D1441146

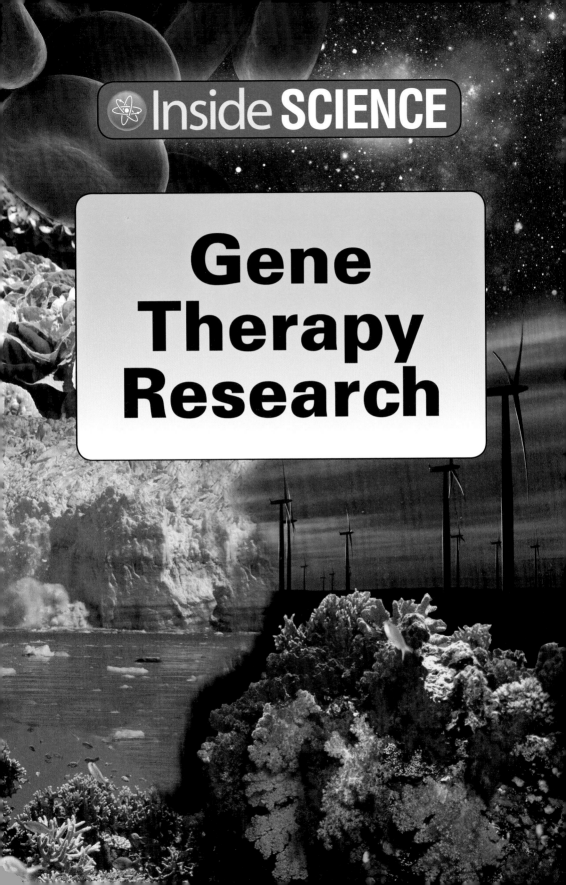

Inside SCIENCE

Gene Therapy Research

Other titles in the *Inside Science* series:

Climate Change Research
Renewable Energy Research
Space Research
Stem Cell Research
Vaccine Research

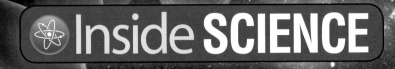

Gene
Therapy
Research

Hal Marcovitz

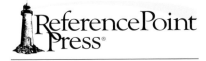

ReferencePoint
Press®

San Diego, CA

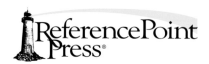

ReferencePoint Press®

© 2011 ReferencePoint Press, Inc.

For more information, contact:
ReferencePoint Press, Inc.
PO Box 27779
San Diego, CA 92198
www.ReferencePointPress.com

LIBRARY OF CONGRESS CATALOGING-IN-PUBLICATION DATA

Marcovitz, Hal.
  Gene therapy research / by Hal Marcovitz.
      p. cm. — (Inside science)
  Includes bibliographical references and index.
  ISBN-13: 978-1-60152-108-8 (hardback)
  ISBN-10: 1-60152-108-1 (hardback)
  1. Gene therapy—Research. I. Title.
  RB155.8.M37 2009
  615.8'95—dc22

                                                                              2009041686

Contents

Foreword

I n 2008, when the Yale Project on Climate Change and the George Mason University Center for Climate Change Communication asked Americans, "Do you think that global warming is happening?" 71 percent of those polled—a significant majority—answered "yes." When the poll was repeated in 2010, only 57 percent of respondents said they believed that global warming was happening. Other recent polls have reported a similar shift in public opinion about climate change.

Although respected scientists and scientific organizations worldwide warn that a buildup of greenhouse gases, mainly caused by human activities, is bringing about potentially dangerous and long-term changes in Earth's climate, it appears that doubt is growing among the general public. What happened to bring about this change in attitude over such a short period of time? Climate change skeptics claim that scientists have greatly overstated the degree and the dangers of global warming. Others argue that powerful special interests are minimizing the problem for political gain. Unlike experiments conducted under strictly controlled conditions in a lab or petri dish, scientific theories, facts, and findings on such a critical topic as climate change are often subject to personal, political, and media bias—whether for good or for ill.

At its core, however, scientific research is not about politics or 30-second sound bites. Scientific research is about questions and measurable observations. Science is the process of discovery and the means for developing a better understanding of ourselves and the world around us. Science strives for facts and conclusions unencumbered by bias, distortion, and political sensibilities. Although sometimes the methods and motivations are flawed, science attempts to develop a body of knowledge that can guide decision makers, enhance daily life, and lay a foundation to aid future generations.

The relevance and the implications of scientific research are profound, as members of the National Academy of Sciences point out in the 2009 edition of *On Being a Scientist: A Guide to Responsible Conduct in Research*:

Some scientific results directly affect the health and well-being of individuals, as in the case of clinical trials or toxicological studies. Science also is used by policy makers and voters to make informed decisions on such pressing issues as climate change, stem cell research, and the mitigation of natural hazards. . . . And even when scientific results have no immediate applications—as when research reveals new information about the universe or the fundamental constituents of matter—new knowledge speaks to our sense of wonder and paves the way for future advances.

The *Inside Science* series provides students with a sense of the painstaking work that goes into scientific research—whether its focus is microscopic cells cultured in a lab or planets far beyond the solar system. Each book in the series examines how scientists work and where that work leads them. Sometimes, the results are positive. Such was the case for Edwin McClure, a once-active high school senior diagnosed with multiple sclerosis, a degenerative disease that leads to difficulties with coordination, speech, and mobility. Thanks to stem cell therapy, in 2009 a symptom-free McClure strode across a stage to accept his diploma from Virginia Commonwealth University. In some cases, cutting-edge experimental treatments fail with tragic results. This is what occurred in 1999 when 18-year-old Jesse Gelsinger, born with a rare liver disease, died four days after undergoing a newly developed gene therapy technique. Such failures may temporarily halt research, as happened in the Gelsinger case, to allow for investigation and revision. In this and other instances, however, research resumes, often with renewed determination to find answers and solve problems.

Through clear and vivid narrative, carefully selected anecdotes, and direct quotations each book in the *Inside Science* series reinforces the role of scientific research in advancing knowledge and creating a better world. By developing an understanding of science, the responsibilities of the scientist, and how scientific research affects society, today's students will be better prepared for the critical challenges that await them. As members of the National Academy of Sciences state: "The values on which science is based—including honesty, fairness, collegiality, and openness—serve as guides to action in everyday life as well as in research. These values have helped produce a scientific enterprise of unparalleled usefulness, productivity, and creativity. So long as these values are honored, science—and the society it serves—will prosper."

Important Events in Gene Therapy Research

1869
Johannes Friedrich Miescher identifies nucleic acids in the bodies of living things, of which deoxyribonucleic acid, DNA, is one.

1902
Archibald Garrod provides scientific proof that not all diseases are contracted through exposure to viruses or bacteria and that some are inherited.

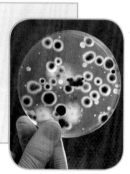

1859
Charles Darwin publishes *On the Origin of Species* stating his theories on evolution, including the evolution of diseases.

1840   **1880**   **1920**   **1960**

1895
German zoologist Valentin Häcker withdraws undifferentiated cells from the very young embryo of an aquatic animal. He uses the term *Stammzelle*—in English, "stem cell"—to describe the cells.

1926
Hermann J. Muller determines the gene is the carrier of biological information.

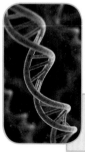

1944
Oswald Avery and Maclyn McCarty identify DNA, the chemical found in all genes, as the agent of hereditary.

1953
Francis Crick and James D. Watson discover the structure of DNA, identifying it as a complex and twisted ladder they label the "double helix."

1961
Crick establishes a link between DNA and disease when he finds DNA provides the instructions for the manufacture of proteins, which carry out all functions of the body.

IMPORTANT EVENTS

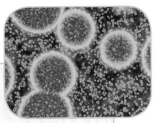

2002
A virus used to deliver new genes to three French children turns on dormant genes in their bodies, causing them to develop blood cancer; two of the children recover but one dies.

1973
Stanley Cohen and Herbert Boyer perform the first gene transfer, inserting a new gene into an *E. coli* bacterium.

1999
In an experiment at the University of Pennsylvania in Philadelphia, gene therapy patient Jesse Gelsinger dies after his immune system reacts to the virus carrying the new genes.

2003
Competing public and private projects announce completion of the Human Genome Project, which maps some 23,000 genes found in the human species.

1983
In an experiment on mice, researchers at Baylor University in Texas replace faulty genes with healthy genes.

1970　　**1980**　　**1990**　　**2000**　　**2010**

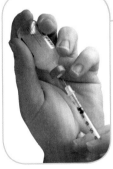

1982
American drug companies begin manufacturing insulin, a chemical needed by diabetes patients, by genetically altering bacteria.

2000
The U.S. Food and Drug Administration (FDA) announces tough new guidelines for laboratories pursuing gene therapies, including random inspections by FDA officials.

2009
Drug companies prepare to release an antimalaria drug created through synthetic biology—the use of DNA as building blocks to create new organisms.

1990
Ashanthi DeSilva is the first human to receive gene replacement therapy; doctors treat her severe combined immunodeficiency by injecting the young girl with new genes that are carried in a virus.

2005
Genetic tests reveal how certain drugs fail to work in the bodies of some cancer patients.

Replacing Faulty Genes

Researchers at University College London in Great Britain have employed an experimental therapy on a dozen youths born with a condition known as Leber's congenital amaurosis, or LCA, which robs patients of their eyesight as they grow older. LCA is caused by a faulty gene that inhibits the production of an enzyme, which is a chemical that causes a reaction in the body. This enzyme promotes the growth of new photoreceptor cells in the backs of the eyes, but people who suffer from LCA lack the enzyme, and therefore their eyes are unable to produce new photoreceptor cells.

> **genes**
>
> Basic biological units of heredity. Genes are composed of DNA, which determines the characteristics that make up every living creature.

The job of the photoreceptor cells is to accept light through the iris, then transmit the light to the brain, which forms the image of what the eye sees. Without production of the enzyme, existing photoreceptor cells gradually die off, and patients with LCA slowly lose their eyesight. By their teenage years, most LCA patients find they have trouble seeing in dimly lit conditions; they usually experience total blindness by the time they are young adults.

The Genetic Culprit

The culprit is the faulty gene, which scientists have labeled RPE65. Genes are very tiny components of virtually all cells found in living things. They provide the building blocks of life; these building blocks determine all of the characteristics that make up each individual person. Genes determine whether a person has brown hair or blue eyes, whether a person will be short or tall, thin or obese, or whether a person will develop certain diseases or debilitations, including some that cause blindness.

Using gene therapy, doctors at University College injected healthy copies of RPE65 into the eyes of the dozen British teens. Since receiving the therapy in 2007, each of the nearly blind teenagers has shown dramatic improvement. Before Steven Howarth received the therapy, researchers filmed him trying to make his way through a dimly lit maze. The film shows Howarth bumping into walls as he struggles to find his way through the corridors. It took the young patient 77 seconds to feel his way through the maze and find the exit.

Howarth then received injections of RPE65. Six months later, Howarth walked through the same maze. He found his way out of the maze

Brice Mellen of Lincoln, Nebraska, is blind because of a condition known as Leber's congenital amaurosis (LCA). An experimental form of gene therapy has given the gift of sight to some LCA patients.

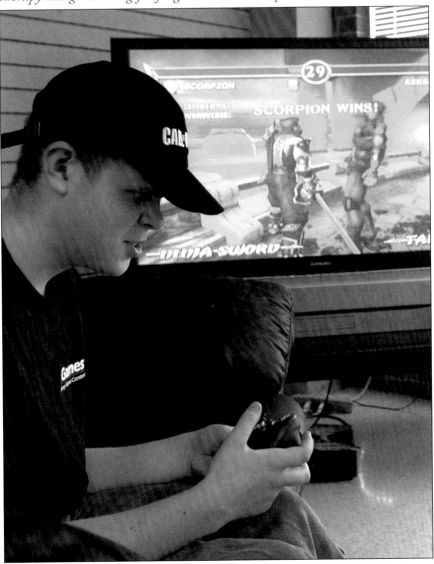

in just 14 seconds and had no difficulty negotiating through the dimly lit corridors. "I don't have any doubt this is going to be a real home run," says Jeffrey Boatright, a gene therapy researcher at Emory University in Atlanta, Georgia. "The people in this trial, they're going to be out playing Frisbee, seeing their girlfriends' and boyfriends' faces for the first time."[1]

Tremendous Potential of Gene Therapy

The treatments performed on Howarth and the other young British patients illustrate the tremendous potential of gene therapy. Faulty genes are responsible for as many as 4,000 diseases and debilitations that afflict tens of millions of patients. Among these genetically related diseases are sickle-cell anemia, hemophilia, cystic fibrosis, and many forms of cancer. Patients do not contract these illnesses through exposure to viruses or bacteria. Rather, the diseases are hardwired into their DNA.

> **enzyme**
>
> Chemical composed of protein that drives a reaction in the body; missing or faulty enzymes often cause diseases and debilitations.

All of these conditions and others are inherited from their parents or other close relatives—just as they inherit hair color and height. As such, they have no natural defenses against contracting these diseases.

In recent years, though, researchers have started perfecting therapies to treat these maladies. As in the case of the LCA patients in Great Britain, doctors have found that by manipulating the genetic makeup of the patients, they can neutralize the genes that cause disease and offer cures that a generation ago were regarded as unthinkable. "The number of potential beneficiaries is awesome," write authors Jeff Lyon and Peter Gorner in their book *Altered Fates: Gene Therapy and the Retooling of Human Life.*

> While only a small fraction, perhaps 15 percent, of the public suffers from the rarer forms of genetic disorders, the percentage of those affected swells hugely if one takes into account maladies that appear later in life, such as cancer, cardiovascular disorder, Alzheimer's disease, depression, and diabetes. Heart and other circulatory ailments affect more than two million people in the United States each year, and cancer afflicts a million more. Together, they are responsible for nearly a million and a half deaths a year, or approximately 75 percent of all deaths.[2]

Moreover, the science of gene research goes beyond simply replacing bad genes with good genes. In recent years scientists have been able to develop drugs that turn off bad genes that cause disease. They have developed techniques to genetically test patients to find out whether the drugs they are taking are effective. They have found ways to inject genetic material into very young cells that grow into healthy cells, replacing diseased cells in patients. And they have developed technology that employs devices small enough to detect genes that cause cancer. All of these advancements have been made possible because scientists have gained a better understanding of the human genome.

Emboldened by Success

Meanwhile, the type of gene replacement therapy received by the British LCA patients is very new—the first patient to receive a similar gene therapy was treated in 1990. Doctors have had just 20 years to evaluate the therapy, assess the results, and improve their techniques. Many mysteries about gene therapy remain, meaning that some ill effects may yet manifest themselves. That is why many physicians, political leaders, and other experts have urged doctors and their patients to proceed with caution. And that is also why the U.S. Food and Drug Administration (FDA), which approves all medicinal therapies in America, has yet to authorize a single form of gene replacement therapy for widespread use.

Indeed, some critics believe gene therapy may be a waste of time and resources and that the billions of dollars spent on the science could be better used in other areas of medical research. Horace Freeland Judson, a science historian at George Washington University in Washington, D.C., argues that no two genetic diseases are alike, and therefore the research is enormously complicated and likely to

photoreceptor cells

Found in the back of the eye, cells that transmit light to the brain, which then forms an image of what the eye sees.

produce few positive results. "Because these diseases have different genetic causes and affect different types of tissue, each presents a new set of research problems to be solved almost from scratch," he says. "As the millions [of dollars] burned away, it became clear that even with success, the cost per patient would continue to be enormous. And success has shown itself just beyond reach. . . . From the start, step by step, everybody has

human genome

The total genetic information contained in the human body.

underestimated the real difficulties the science presents."[3]

Still, gene therapy researchers press on, emboldened by the results shown in the British LCA cases as well as other success stories that have recently surfaced. Says Robin Ali, the gene therapy researcher who headed the British LCA study, "Moving something from the laboratory to the clinic, the difficulty of doing that is enormous. It's very exciting that we've managed to get this far."[4]

What Is Gene Therapy?

In simple terms, gene therapy is the use of genes as medicine. A main focus of gene therapy is the replacement of faulty genes with healthy genes, although in some cases the healthy genes are used to repair or "turn off" the faulty genes. "It's basically a transplant,"[5] says Stuart Orkin, a Harvard University physician who has pioneered gene therapy. Instead of transplanting a faulty heart with a healthy heart or a failing kidney with a functioning kidney, physicians replace faulty genes with healthy genes, which are among the tiniest parts of human anatomy.

Genes and DNA

Genes are components of threadlike structures known as chromosomes. Nearly every human cell contains 46 chromosomes in 23 matching pairs—one chromosome in each pair is inherited from the mother, one from the father. Each chromosome includes strings of genes. Genes are composed of deoxyribonucleic acid, or DNA, the molecule found in virtually every cell of every living thing on Earth. DNA includes every characteristic that makes up the person, chimpanzee, dog, cat, earthworm, beetle, stalk of celery, blade of grass, or ear of corn. The DNA found in each gene contains the information that determines the characteristics living things inherit from their parents. Each human body is estimated to contain about 23,000 genes.

The DNA that is passed on from generation to generation decides the colors of a person's hair and eyes, whether that person is short or tall, thin or stout. If a father has lost his hair at a young age, then his son may also be looking forward to a receding hairline. Athletic ability can be an inherited trait—that is why the sons and daughters of many professional athletes grow into superb athletes themselves: Their raw athletic talent and physiques have been inherited from their parents. Intelligence can also be an inherited trait. So are freckles.

And so are many diseases and debilitations. People have inherited such minor annoyances as color blindness and skin blemishes from their parents, grandparents, or great-grandparents (it is not unusual for traits to skip generations before making themselves known) as well as some truly devastating conditions such as Alzheimer's disease, which robs people of their memories, and Down syndrome, which impedes the mental and physical growth of those afflicted. Many medical researchers believe that gene therapy holds the key to potentially curing all debilitating conditions that patients inherit from their parents and other relatives. "There is

The threadlike structures called chromosomes (pictured in a computer illustration) consist of strings of genes composed of DNA tightly coiled many times around proteins. Nearly every human cell contains 46 chromosomes in 23 matching pairs.

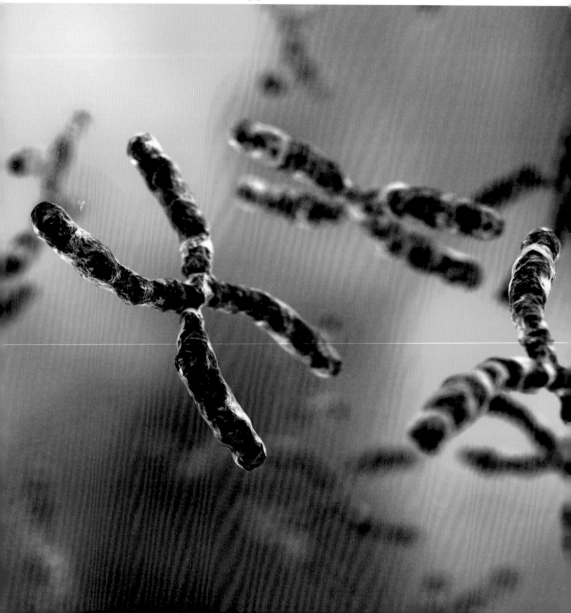

a growing sense that with molecular biology in general and gene therapy in particular all things are possible,"[6] write Lyon and Gorner.

In many inherited diseases and debilitations, the reaction of the body's 2 million proteins to the bad genes often results in pain, illness, and disability. Gene therapy is designed to make proteins act normally. This science is known as proteomics—the study of proteins, particularly the genetic structure of proteins. (The term *proteomics* is a combination of the words *protein* and *genome*.) The human body also contains about 75,000 enzymes. These are substances composed of proteins that drive chemical reactions in the body—or, in the case of disease, are missing or otherwise fail to perform their tasks. Scientists believe that faulty proteins and missing enzymes can be fixed by replacing the genes that are ultimately at the root of the mischief, but replacing bad genes with healthy genes is still regarded as highly experimental.

> ## chromosomes
>
> Threadlike structures found in most cells in living things; humans normally have 46 chromosomes, 23 inherited from each parent. Each chromosome is composed of a series of genes.

How People Inherit Diseases

Gene therapy can trace its roots to the work of Charles Darwin, the British naturalist whose *On the Origin of Species*, published in 1859, established the concept that physical traits are passed down from generation to generation. Darwin's work enraged many people who believed strongly in the biblical explanation for the creation of the human race and rejected the notion that people evolved from lower forms of life. Sparking far less controversy at the time were Darwin's theories about diseases as well as physical and mental disabilities—that they, too, were inherited from one's parents. "There are many . . . diseases, which are not attached to any particular period, but which certainly tend to appear in the child at about the same age at which the parent was first attacked,"[7] Darwin wrote. In his work, Darwin discusses one case in particular: "Two brothers, their father, their paternal uncles, seven cousins, and their paternal grandfather, were all similarly affected by a skin-disease, called pityriasis versicolor; the disease, strictly limited to the males in the family (though transmitted through the females), usually appeared at puberty, and disappeared at about the age of 40 or 45 years."[8]

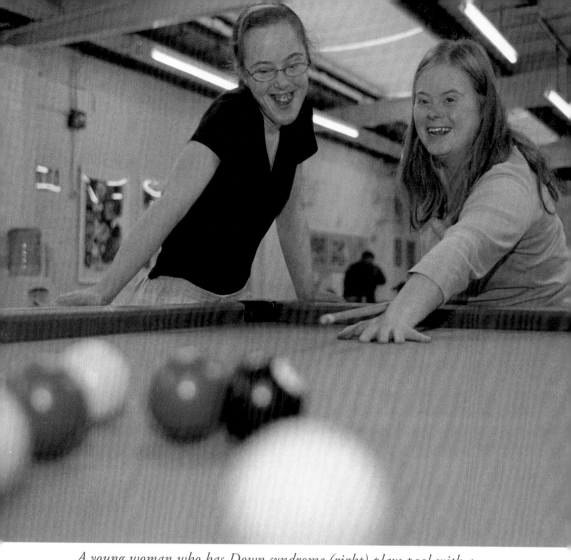

A young woman who has Down syndrome (right) plays pool with a friend. Down syndrome results from a chromosomal abnormality. Medical researchers believe that gene therapy holds the key to curing or preventing inherited conditions such as this one.

Pityriasis versicolor is a mild disease of the skin that manifests itself in white blotches which, as Darwin notes, mostly go away as the patients grow older. As Darwin suggests, the disease is believed to have a genetic element, passed down from generation to generation.

Darwin's work is regarded as an important milestone in establishing the inherited qualities of many diseases, but Darwin was not a doctor, and therefore his work merely cites his own observations and theories and lacks the authority of clinical tests performed by physicians. Soon, though, some doctors would start applying Darwin's principles to their own work and clinical experiences, and they would begin drawing the same conclusions as Darwin about the inherited nature of many diseases.

Indeed, a great step forward occurred in 1902 when the English physician Archibald Garrod examined a patient for back pain and arthritis, a bone disease that mostly affects the joints. The patient also exhibited dark bluish black bruises. The patient provided Garrod with a urine sample, which turned black after a few days. Garrod recognized the disease as alkaptonuria, also known as black urine disease. At the time, it was believed that alkaptonuria was caused by a bacterial infection of the intestine. Moreover, doctors believed the disease was contagious, meaning a patient could catch alkaptonuria from another person. After making inquiries, though, Garrod determined that the disease seemed to run in families.

In an experiment, Garrod fed alkaptonuria patients meals high in protein and observed that the more protein they ate, the darker their urine turned. He found that their bodies lacked an enzyme necessary for them to break down and metabolize proteins, and that the buildup of proteins in their bodies was causing pain, arthritis, the bluish black bruises, and dark urine. Garrod concluded that the lack of the enzyme in their bodies was due to an "inborn error of metabolism"[9]—in other words, they were born without the enzyme. Garrod did not suggest his alkaptonuria patients were lacking a gene that would provide the enzyme, but his work provided scientific proof that some patients inherit diseases and debilitations from their parents.

Exploring the Links Between Genes and Disease

The work by other researchers studying genetics would provide important discoveries in the science. In 1869 Swiss biologist Johannes Friedrich Miescher identified chemicals in blood that he called nuclein—now known as nucleic acids, of which DNA is one. During the 1920s, American Hermann J. Muller established the gene as the carrier of biological information.

Meanwhile, other scientists were exploring the links between genes and diseases. Harvard University Medical School professor William Bosworth Castle studied sickle-cell anemia and found that the disease is caused by abnormal proteins. Sickle-cell anemia is a disease of the blood that can be horrific. In blood that is free of the disease, red blood cells form into doughnut shapes and flow easily through the body's blood

Mutated Genes and Ethnic Groups

Members of the same ethnic groups often trace their ancestries to a common area, which often means they have common ancestors. That is why certain diseases are common among people of the same ethnic group.

Sickle-cell anemia afflicts mostly people who trace their roots to sub-Saharan Africa. In the United States, the disease afflicts mostly African Americans. About 72,000 patients, most of whom are African American, are afflicted with the disease, although it is believed that about 2 million African Americans—about 1 in 12 members of the ethnic group—carry the mutated gene that causes the disease.

Another ethnic group afflicted with a mutated gene includes Jews of eastern and central European descent. Known as Ashkenazi Jews, they often pass on a mutated gene that causes Tay-Sachs disease. The disease is caused by a buildup of a fatty substance in nerve cells and manifests itself in blindness, deafness, and deterioration of mental abilities. Children born with Tay-Sachs eventually suffer from seizures and lose the ability to move their limbs. The disease usually results in death by the age of four.

Screening methods have been able to identify carriers of sickle-cell anemia as well as Tay-Sachs; therefore, couples can be warned about the likelihood that their children will be affected. Still, Tay-Sachs is believed to kill about 30 American children a year, while sickle-cell anemia takes about 500 American lives a year.

vessels. In blood afflicted with sickle-cell anemia, the red blood cells curve, forming into shapes that resemble sickles (agricultural tools used to reap crops). The sickle-shaped cells do not move easily through the vessels—they are stiff and sticky and form into clumps, which limits blood flow. People who suffer from sickle-cell anemia experience pain, organ damage, and infections because parts of their bodies are starved for blood.

Chemist Linus Pauling pursued research into sickle-cell anemia further, finding that proteins are composed of molecules known as amino acids and that amino acids form into strings that create proteins. Later, scientists concluded that amino acids are linked together by another nucleic acid—ribonucleic acid, or RNA, which is a duplicate of the DNA spawned by the gene. Therefore, a mutated gene produces a mutated form of RNA, which produces faulty strings of amino acids and, therefore, bad proteins that could lead to diseases and debilitations.

Meanwhile, English biochemist Frederick Sanger was able to break down the chemical composition of a protein known as insulin, an important chemical that enables the body to burn sugar as an energy source. Sanger's work showed that insulin is composed of a unique sequence of amino acids. Further, his work showed that when the sequence is faulty—when the sequence may be missing an amino acid—the result could have a devastating impact on the human body. In sickle-cell anemia, for example, the missing amino acids cause the blood cells to sickle.

Finding the Secret of Life

Given the information contained in proteins as well as their importance in the makeup of the human body, researchers found themselves suspecting that proteins are manufactured by genes and that genes are composed of DNA. In 1944 Americans Oswald Avery and Maclyn McCarty determined that DNA is the agent of heredity. And in 1953 a landmark paper was published by James D. Watson, a biologist, and Francis Crick, a chemist, who determined that DNA molecules are composed of two strands resembling a twisted ladder—the so-called double helix. This was a significant discovery—before the work by Watson and Crick, researchers assumed DNA was a relatively simple molecule, but the two scientists showed its enormous complexity, making it clear that DNA molecules contain voluminous amounts of information about the human body and how that information is passed on from generation to generation. Soon after making the discovery, Crick is said to have walked into a pub around the corner from the lab at Cambridge University in England and announced to all in attendance, "We have found the secret of life."[10] Eight years later, Crick provided an important link between DNA and disease when he found that DNA contains instructions for the manufacture of the body's proteins—meaning that when genes are faulty they make faulty proteins, and so things could go terribly wrong in the body.

DNA

Also known by its formal name deoxyribonucleic acid, the molecule found in virtually every cell of every living thing on Earth. Found in the shape of a long ladder, or double helix, in humans the molecule consists of four base chemicals that form some 3 billion combinations.

Scientists Refine Their Techniques

Soon, discoveries about the nature and structure of DNA paved the way for scientists to isolate specific genes in cells. In 1973 Stanley Cohen of Stanford University in California and Herbert Boyer of the nearby University of California at San Francisco collaborated on a project to insert a new gene into the bacterium *Escherichia coli*, which is commonly known as *E. coli* and found in the human intestine. For the first time, scientists had used gene therapy to alter the biological makeup of a living thing—albeit, in this case, the recipient of the new gene was nothing more than a microscopic germ. Still, it would not take long for scientists to progress from experimenting on the simplest organisms to much more complex subjects, such as plants, laboratory animals, and, eventually, humans.

> ### proteins
> Chemicals manufactured by genes; when genes are faulty, the proteins they make are often faulty, causing breakdowns in the body.

At Baylor University in Texas, scientists isolated a faulty gene believed to cause Lesch-Nyhan disease, which manifests itself in mental retardation. In 1983, while experimenting on mice, the scientists replaced the faulty gene with a healthy gene. Over the next seven years, scientists refined techniques for isolating individual genes in cells, withdrawing them, and injecting them into laboratory animals to treat inherited diseases and debilitations.

The First Human Patient

In 1990 the first human patient received gene replacement therapy. The patient was four-year-old Ashanthi DeSilva, who was born with a mutant gene that made her body unable to produce adenosine deaminase, or ADA, an enzyme vital to maintaining immunity to disease. Ashanthi suffered from a disease known as severe combined immunodeficiency, or SCID, which is more commonly known as "bubble boy disease."

Without ADA the body is unable to fight off infection. It means that simple infections, such as the common cold, could lead to bouts of pneumonia and other serious, life-threatening diseases. In fact, many patients who lack ADA eventually die at young ages. Bubble boy disease gets its name from the case of David Vetter, an SCID patient who lived most of his life in a plastic room, or bubble, that was sealed off against germs. He died at the age of 12.

By age four, Ashanthi had already battled pneumonia a number of times, and physicians believed that without gene therapy she would die within a few years. Her parents quickly agreed to the experimental therapy. Said her father, Raj DeSilva, "What choice did we have?"[11]

Working at the National Institutes of Health (NIH) in Bethesda, Maryland, physicians withdrew blood from the girl's arm and extracted white blood cells. Those cells were then cultured in the lab. As those cells grew into billions of new cells in a test tube, the doctors added cells that

In people who have sickle-cell anemia, normal doughnut-shaped red blood cells (top) curve into sickle shapes (bottom) as seen in this colored scanning electron micrograph. Studies of sickle-cell anemia helped researchers understand the link between genes and disease.

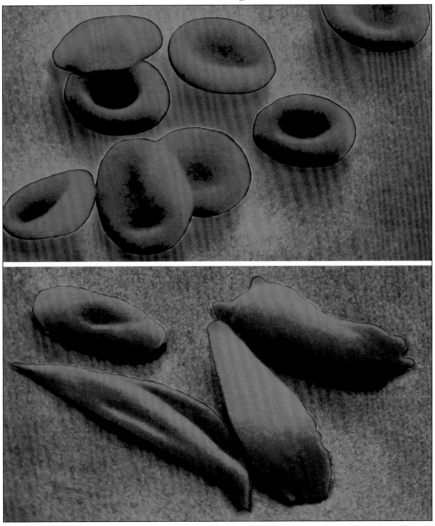

included normal ADA genes. It sounds like a simple procedure, but, in fact, the project took the talents of nearly 100 physicians, nurses, biologists, and other medical personnel. Moreover, the project's leaders had to convince the FDA of the safety of the procedure—the doctors were, after all, about to perform a highly experimental medical procedure on a four-year-old girl. Certainly, the FDA as well as Ashanthi's doctors had many reasons to be concerned—mostly, they worried that the new cells would turn malignant, essentially growing into a cancer in Ashanthi's blood. W. French Anderson, the lead physician in the experiment, recalled the nightmares that kept him awake as the day of Ashanthi's experimental therapy approached: "I saw her gasping and dying in bed. . . . Gene therapy would have been set back years, perhaps indefinitely."[12]

Saving Ashanti

Finally, after months of discussions with the FDA, the federal agency gave its approval, and the DeSilvas were summoned to Bethesda from their home in suburban Cleveland, Ohio. At a few minutes before 1 o'clock in the afternoon on September 14, 1990, as Ashanthi watched the Disney movie *Dumbo* on a hospital TV, the cultured white blood cells were injected back into the little girl's arm. This history-making procedure took about 30 minutes.

The injection on that first day was only the first of many that Ashanthi would receive as part of her gene replacement treatments. Over the next several months, the Bethesda doctors monitored their patient closely. Ashanthi not only survived the therapy but has thrived, growing into an active young woman who plays piano and basketball and rarely comes down with a cold. She appears to have no trouble fighting off infections. Says Anderson, "Ashi is now a delightful young lady. She leads a totally normal life, and she's grown up."[13]

The Ashanthi DeSilva case is very much an unfinished story. She is not believed to be "cured" of the genetic deficiency that makes her body unable to produce its own ADA. Rather, she undergoes regular injections of the healthy genes. Doctors fear that if they cease the treatments, her

RNA

Also known by its formal name, ribonucleic acid, the chemical that links together amino acids, which form proteins. If spawned by a faulty gene, faulty RNA could lead to development of a faulty protein, resulting in disease.

Archibald Garrod

The first physician to recognize the hereditary nature of some diseases was Archibald Garrod, who was born in 1857 in London, England. Although he was the son of a physician, Garrod at first did not plan to follow his father into medicine. He studied art, geography, astronomy, and natural science before deciding to enter medical school. He was soon drawn to the study of chemistry and disease.

He made his breakthrough while treating a patient for alkaptonuria. Refusing to accept the theory that the disease is caused by bacteria, Garrod studied the case histories of 31 patients and concluded that alkaptonuria seemed to run in families. Indeed, one of his patients, whom he identified as Thomas P., shared the malady with two siblings. The theory earned considerable weight when Garrod learned that Thomas P.'s parents were cousins. It meant that two members of a family, who had married each other, evidently passed the disease on to their three children.

Garrod went on to identify other diseases as hereditary, most notably porphyria and albinism. Porphyria is caused by a defective protein and is believed to have led to the insanity of the English monarch George III. Albinism prevents the body from manufacturing the pigment melanin, which gives color to skin.

body will revert to its prior state and lose its immunity to infection. That is why doctors concede that regardless of the promise shown by gene therapy, the treatments are still in the experimental phase and not yet ready for widespread use. Moreover, some scientists predict it could be decades before gene therapies are as common as shots of penicillin. Still, they are optimistic that gene therapy can become a routine procedure available for a variety of illnesses. Says Anderson, "There will be gene-based treatment for essentially every disease, within 50 years."[14]

Mapping the Human Genome

As Ashanthi was receiving her new genes in Bethesda, a separate project was just getting under way that would soon provide an important new tool for gene therapists—specifically, a map of every gene in the human species. This map would help doctors determine which genes are likely to spark diseases and debilitations and how these genes could be turned on or turned off.

Known as the Human Genome Project, the map was completed in 2003 and provided doctors with information on some 23,000 genes found in human anatomy. Even before the mapping was finished, the project showed results: Scientists announced discoveries of genes responsible for causing deafness, epilepsy, asthma, diabetes, and migraine headaches.

Two separate groups of scientists worked on the map—not in co-operation but in competition. One team was funded by the National Institutes of Health, the other by a private company, Celera Genomics, which realized the enormous commercial potential of providing drug companies with a map of the human genome. Such information could help drug companies develop medications to fix or replace faulty genes. "The text [of the genome] is filled with long-sought answers, some amazing surprises, puzzling mysteries, and lots of useful information for medicine,"[15] said Eric Lander, a Massachusetts Institute of Technology biologist who worked on the NIH project.

Before the mapping projects started, researchers already knew that the twisted ladder of DNA—the double helix—is made up of four so-called "base chemicals": adenine, which is abbreviated as A; guanine, G; cytosine, C; and thymine, T. In every DNA molecule—and therefore in every gene—these chemicals form bonds and pair up, creating potentially some 3 billion pairs. The map of the human genome showed scientists how these chemicals fit together in each rung of the double helix, deciding whether a person has brown hair or blonde hair or blue eyes or hazel eyes or whether he or she will be tall or short, thin

adenosine deaminase

Also known as ADA, an enzyme vital to maintaining immunity to disease.

or stocky. And the sequences of A, G, C, and T also determine whether a person will one day develop Alzheimer's disease, many forms of cancer, and other inherited diseases.

These four chemicals switch on proteins. Therefore, by mapping the human genome, the researchers have helped doctors recognize the chemical properties of genes that prompt proteins to break down or otherwise act incorrectly, causing diseases and debilitations. Said Francis Collins, head of the NIH project,

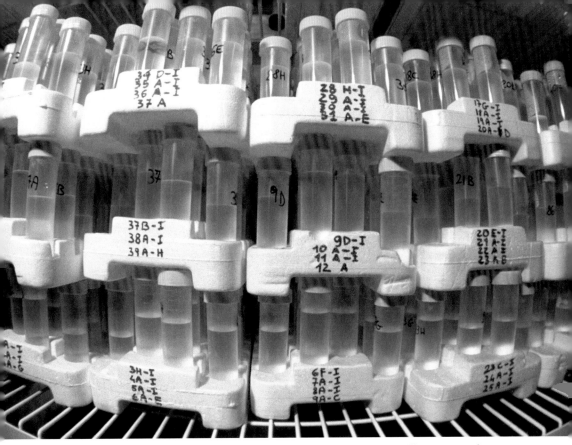

Test tubes containing samples of DNA found in human cells are stored in a laboratory. Samples such as these were used in the Human Genome Project, which mapped all of the genes found in the human anatomy.

For me as a physician, as somebody who is really interested in tracking down the genes that contribute to disease—to heart disease, to colon cancer, to diabetes, to Alzheimer's disease—it means that the number of genes we have to deal with and sift through is a shorter list. And that's good news. That means we should be able to find the ones we're most interested in, somewhat more easily. Our haystack isn't quite as big as we feared it would be. That should advance the rate of progress in the medical consequences of this project, which is really the reason to do it."[16]

Still an Experimental Therapy

As the work of Garrod, Watson, Crick, and the scientists who labored over the Human Genome Project illustrate, new breakthroughs in gene therapy provide scientists with a deep understanding of the role of genes in human diseases. Scientists are just beginning to apply that knowledge to treating human patients. The highly experimental nature of the therapy means it may be decades before the FDA approves gene therapy on a widespread basis. Still, as the success of the Ashanthi DeSilva case proves, gene therapy has the potential for curing illnesses that are otherwise believed to be incurable.

The Ideal Gene-Delivery Vehicle: Viruses

When doctors at the National Institutes of Health injected new genes into the arm of Ashanthi DeSilva, they could not simply load up a hypodermic needle with good genes and inject them right into the little girl's bloodstream. The genes had to be able to penetrate Ashanthi's white blood cells, where they could implant the DNA that produces adenosine deaminase and thereby bolster her immune system.

The doctors needed a Trojan horse—in other words, a vehicle to carry the hidden genes through the otherwise impenetrable cellular walls, just as the ancient Greeks built a wooden horse, then hid inside as their enemies, the Trojans, pulled the horse through the gates of their city. The answer turned out to be simple: They used a virus—similar to the germ that causes colds or flu—to carry the genes and break through the cell walls.

Viruses as Vectors

Viruses have turned out to be effective Trojan horses. (Scientists prefer to call them vectors.) For starters, they are very good at breaking through cell walls—that is how they carry out their infections, causing people to catch colds and flu or other more serious diseases. Once they penetrate the cell walls, viruses plant their own genes inside the cells, so it seemed logical that if the viruses were first implanted with genes that could cure diseases, the viruses would plant those genes in the recipient cells as well. Says W. French Anderson, the lead physician in Ashanthi's gene therapy, "Because it's a human virus—many of us have [viruses] in our throats all the time . . . it's able to get into a broad range of cell types."[17]

In Ashanthi's case, the viral vector delivered the genes and successfully cured her of SCID, which would probably have been fatal without gene therapy. Not all gene therapies employing viruses have been as successful as the technique used to treat Ashanthi. In some cases, the viruses turn out to be poor carriers and have failed to deliver the genes effectively. In other cases, the viruses have turned malevolent, causing serious illness rather than providing cures. Indeed, in one case a patient's severely adverse reaction to a virus prompted government regulators to take a hard look at whether the risks of using viruses are worth the benefits that gene therapy has promised to deliver.

Billions of Copies

Viruses make ideal vectors because, by their nature, they are infectious. The typical virus consists of its own DNA contained in an envelope composed of a protein. Genetic researchers have found they can alter the genetic composition of the virus, stripping away its harmful qualities while adding the healthy genes they want to deliver to the patient.

Once the genetic makeup of the virus has been altered, it is mixed with the patient's white blood cells in a laboratory dish. The virus duplicates itself into billions of copies, which attach themselves to the patient's white blood cells, injecting the genetic material into the cells. These cells are then injected into the patient, where the duplication process continues. "You can do spectacular things with cells in a laboratory dish," says Anderson. "You can easily get the genes in, change the cell's properties and do other things that ought to enable you to treat disease successfully."[18] In fact, the concept of employing viruses to deliver new DNA dates back to the earliest genetic experiments. In 1959 University of Tennessee physician Stanfield Rogers published a paper suggesting that a virus common in rabbits was responsible for decreasing the levels of an amino acid known as arginine in the blood of scientists who had experimented with the rabbits years before. Essentially, Rogers said, the doctors caught the virus from the rabbits; these germs transferred their DNA into the humans, with the result being a lower than normal level of an amino acid in their blood. (Arginine helps keep blood vessels open, which means it is an important chemical for maintaining heart health. Despite catching this rabbit virus, evidently these scientists felt no ill effects from the lower levels of arginine in their bodies.)

> **vectors**
>
> The packages that deliver the gene to the cell. Typically, a virus is used as a vector because of its infectious nature—it attaches itself to the cell, then injects DNA into the cell.

Using HIV as a Vector

One of the most effective viruses that can be employed to transfer genetic material to cells is the human immunodeficiency virus (HIV), which is the virus that causes acquired immune deficiency syndrome (AIDS). Since AIDS can often be a horrific and fatal disease, researchers have been hesitant to use HIV for gene therapy. Still, because the virus is so aggressive, its capability of transferring genes to human cells has long intrigued genetic researchers.

Scientists at the University of California at Los Angeles (UCLA) believe they have neutralized the dangerous features of HIV and have used it as a vector to treat breast cancer in mice. To perform the treatment, the researchers altered the virus to include a cancer-curing gene. "People might wonder if it's scary to use HIV as a therapy," said UCLA genetics researcher Irvin Chen. "In actuality, we have completely removed 80 percent of the virus. So really it's just a carrier." Despite their success, the UCLA researchers remain wary of using HIV in humans and plan many more trials on mice before starting clinical trials on human patients.

Quoted in Kristen Philipkoski, "Altered HIV Attacks Mice Tumors," *Wired*, February 14, 2005. www.wired.com.

By the 1980s, scientists were using viruses to deliver genes to plants, genetically engineering the plants to better resist freezing, pests, and other agricultural hazards. Indeed, the genetic engineering of farm crops has turned into a separate and booming science as food production companies seek ways to improve the taste and resiliency of crops.

Meanwhile, laboratory animals were also getting new genes delivered in viral packages. In 1983 researchers successfully employed a virus that causes leukemia in mice to deliver a gene that can correct hemophilia, a blood disease that often causes uncontrollable bleeding. Before injecting the hemophiliac mice with the virus, the researchers stripped out its disease-causing qualities. So the mice were not being infected with leukemia, which is a cancer of the blood, but merely a shell of a germ that could no longer cause the disease. Other experiments on lab animals followed, and in 1990 Anderson and his colleagues at the NIH were ready for a human test. They applied to the FDA for permission to use a virus to carry the new genes into Ashanthi's body. In Ashanthi's case, the NIH doctors used a leukemia virus to deliver the new genes. As with the mice, prior to the therapy, the malignant features of the leukemia virus were stripped out so that Ashanthi would not develop cancer of the blood.

Risks of Using Viruses

After the success in the Ashanthi DeSilva case, gene therapy moved forward as universities and private labs explored experimental procedures, most of which included the employment of viruses to deliver the genes. Still, many doctors recognized the risks of using viruses as vectors. For example, once a person has been exposed to a virus, that person develops a level of immunity and cannot be affected by that virus again. In gene therapy, many doctors saw the likelihood that the first injection of the viruses could be effective but that, due to the patient's natural powers of immunity, subsequent injections of the vectors would likely have no beneficial effect. Said James M. Wilson, director of the Institute for Human Gene Therapy at the University of Pennsylvania in Philadelphia, "In a very unfortunate turn of events, the patients would become immune against the therapy."[19]

Moreover, doctors were concerned about other reactions of the body's immune system to the introduction of a virus. What if the body's natural immunity—its antibodies—attacked the viruses just as it would attack viruses carrying colds and flu? In fact, in many cases doctors noticed that after injecting their gene therapy patients with vectors, symptoms of redness and swelling would occur at the point of injection—a sure sign that the body's antibodies had been summoned and were now fighting the virus. As Wilson and his colleagues at the University of Pennsylvania lab were soon to discover, one of their patients would suffer an immune reaction to a virus, and in his case the reaction would manifest itself in symptoms much worse than redness and swelling.

metabolize

Process by which a particular substance is handled in the body.

The Tragic Case of Jesse Gelsinger

Jesse Gelsinger, an 18-year-old from Tucson, Arizona, suffered from a rare liver disease known as ornithine transcarbamylase disorder, or OTD. The disease is caused by a faulty gene that prevents the body from metabolizing ammonia. People are familiar with ammonia as a household cleaner, but it is a rather common chemical found in the environment in many places—even in food (because farmers often use ammonia-based

How Viruses Work

Gene researchers are using viruses to carry healthy genes into cells that contain problem genes. What makes this possible is typical virus behavior. Viruses cannot reproduce on their own. Instead, they invade living "host" cells and then use those cells as factories where they produce more viral material. In this way they spread infection throughout the body. In gene therapy, viruses are used to attack and replace problem genes with healthy ones.

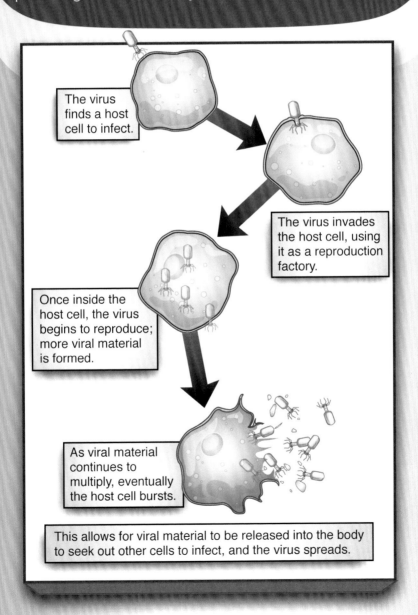

The virus finds a host cell to infect.

The virus invades the host cell, using it as a reproduction factory.

Once inside the host cell, the virus begins to reproduce; more viral material is formed.

As viral material continues to multiply, eventually the host cell bursts.

This allows for viral material to be released into the body to seek out other cells to infect, and the virus spreads.

Source: Craig Freudenrich, "How Viruses Work," How Stuff Works, 2000. http://health.howstuffworks.com.

Shooting DNA with a Gene Gun

Instead of using a virus to break through the wall of a cell, some scientists have experimented with a "gene gun"—a device that would actually shoot DNA into a cell. Gene guns were first used in the 1980s as a method of genetically altering plants. To introduce new genetic material into the plant cell, strands of DNA were first wrapped around microscopic beads of gold, which act like bullets. (Each bead is about a millionth of a meter in diameter.) A blast shoots the gold beads into the plant cells.

The first gene guns were little more than modified electric nail guns used by carpenters, but they have since been constructed specifically for genetic research and use helium or electrical charges to propel the pellets. Most of the research employing gene guns has concentrated on using the technique to inject genetically altered vaccines into the skin cells of patients. In 2009 the University of Alabama at Birmingham commenced a study using the gene gun to inoculate patients with a vaccine to prevent cervical cancer. "The whole technology is so simple," says Harriet L. Robinson, an immunologist at the University of Massachusetts School of Medicine, which has also experimented with a gene gun. "That is the bottom line—it is so simple."

Quoted in David Brown, "Elusive 'Magic Bullet' May Help Shoot Down Infectious Diseases," *Washington Post*, January 10, 1994, p. A-3.

fertilizers on their crops.) Most people metabolize ammonia well, meaning their bodies are able to rid themselves of ammonia by breaking down the chemical and making it harmless, but OTD patients lack the enzyme that enables them to neutralize ammonia. By not being able to break down ammonia, OTD patients are susceptible to severe liver damage. The liver is one of the body's vital organs: Its functions include storing vitamins, sugars, and fats from food, using them to manufacture bodily chemicals. The liver also manufactures bile, which aids in digestion and breaks down substances, such as ammonia, that can harm the body. As an OTD patient, Gelsinger faced a rather bleak future: He was forced to live on a restrictive low-protein diet and also swallow some 50 pills a day to ease his symptoms.

In 1999 Gelsinger learned about a gene therapy program for OTD patients at the University of Pennsylvania. He quickly volunteered for the experimental therapy, even though he and the other 17 volunteers were advised by doctors that the new genes would probably be effective for a few weeks only and that their bodies would soon revert to being unable to metabolize ammonia. Still, Gelsinger was enthusiastic about participating, believing he could help unlock the secrets of curing OTD.

On September 13, 1999, researchers injected healthy genes into Gelsinger's body. They were contained in billions of molecules of the adenovirus—a close cousin of the virus that causes the common cold. Of the 18 participants in the trial, Gelsinger received the highest dose. The vectors carrying the genes were injected into an artery leading directly to the teenager's liver.

Since the researchers believed they had stripped out the virus's malignant features, they were shocked at what happened next: Within hours of the injection, Gelsinger grew gravely ill. Over the next four days, the teenager lost consciousness, and then his organs and other bodily functions failed. Four days after receiving the injection, he died. He is believed to have been the first patient of any form of gene therapy to have been killed by the treatment. "There isn't a day goes by that I don't think about it," says Wilson. "It was humbling for me in many ways, including sort of a realistic reassessment of what we know and don't know . . . I was naïve. The technologies we had available to us at the time were inadequate."[20]

Dangers of Gene Therapy

Clearly, the scientists in the University of Pennsylvania laboratory had not anticipated Gelsinger's reaction to the virus. Although none of the other 17 patients grew ill from the virus, evidently it remained strong enough to spark the severe reaction in Gelsinger's body.

The Gelsinger case prompted government regulators to call a temporary halt to several similar gene therapy research programs while they assessed the safety of the science. Congress held hearings, questioning the techniques used by gene therapy researchers. The University of Pennsylvania sustained a heavy fine from the government as well as a large dose of criticism. Federal investigators found that the university's gene therapy program had been moving too quickly, that Gelsinger was probably too

Viruses make good vectors, carrying healthy genes into the cells, because of how they behave. When an altered virus mixes with the patient's blood, the virus makes billions of copies of itself. The copies then attach to the patient's red blood cells (pictured).

sick to participate in the trial—a year before the trial, he had slipped into a coma due to liver failure—and that in a prior trial staged at the university, laboratory animals administered the adenovirus died during the experiment. In addition, the investigation revealed that the therapy tried on Gelsinger was aimed more at testing the treatment techniques, including the use of the virus, than in curing the teenager's OTD. Said Gelsinger's father, Paul Gelsinger, "Jesse became the poster child for what not to do in human-subjects research."[21]

antibodies

Chemicals found in the blood that are summoned by the body's immune system and dispatched to attack cells carrying disease.

Eventually, research resumed with a lot of resources devoted to finding safer viruses to deliver the genes. At the University of Pennsylvania lab responsible for Gelsinger's death, physicians devoted much of their work to improving the safety of vectors. Since Gelsinger's death, researchers have discovered more than 100 viruses capable of delivering the genes that are considered safer than the virus that killed the teenager. Says Wilson, "I have tremendous regrets about what happened. I feel absolutely awful about what it has done to the family, to this university, to the field."[22]

Still, problems have surfaced. In 2002 three French children treated with gene therapy developed a form of blood cancer similar to leukemia; the virus used to deliver the genes may have activated a dormant cancer gene, essentially turning it on. Two of the children recovered, but one died. The case illustrates one of the true dangers of gene therapy—after the new genes are injected into the body, they may fix the targeted faulty proteins but they may also cause other, unanticipated effects.

Indeed, the genes, or the viruses that carry them, may turn other genes on or off, which could cause a breakdown in other proteins. Doctors have compared the effect to that of the cue ball on a billiards table—the cue ball usually hits the targeted ball, but what happens if the cue ball ricochets and hits other balls as well? They may bounce

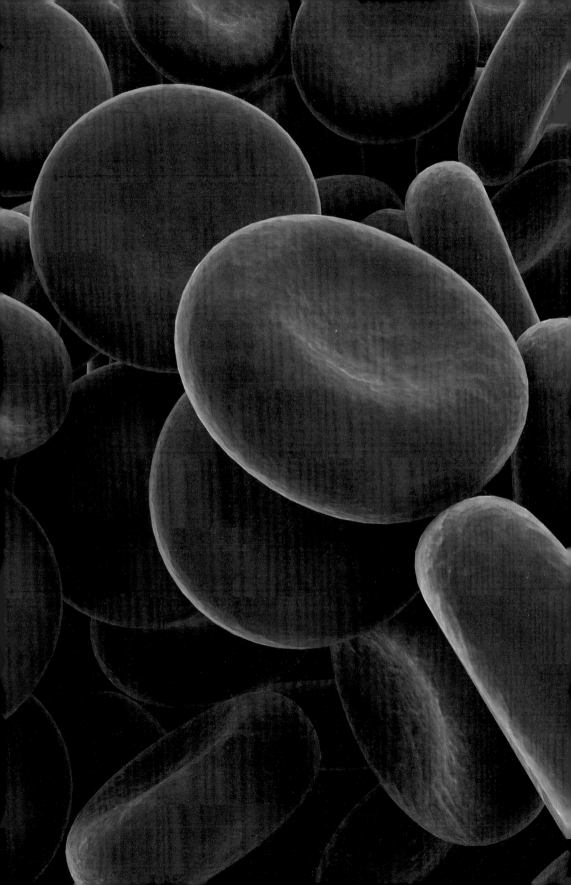

around the table and end up in places the player does not expect. "It's sort of potentially rather bad news for gene therapy because you're hitting just what you'd rather not be hitting,"[23] said Frederick Bushman, a gene therapy researcher at the Salk Institute for Biological Studies in La Jolla, California.

Fixing the Abuses in Human Trials

Soon after the death of Jesse Gelsinger, the FDA launched investigations of all gene therapy trials in the United States and came to some shocking conclusions: Many gene therapy scientists had not been following FDA rules requiring them to report adverse effects of their experiments.

The agency moved quickly, shutting down gene therapy experiments on human subjects at the University of Pennsylvania and also temporarily suspending gene therapy work at other institutions that it found were not following the rules. These included Tufts University in Boston and Schering-Plough Corporation, a New Jersey drug company.

A year after Gelsinger's death, the FDA and NIH announced a new initiative to police human trials in gene therapy: the Gene Therapy Clinical Monitoring Plan. The main feature of the program includes random inspections of labs conducting gene therapy experiments. Said Philip Noguchi, an official of the FDA's Center for Biologics Evaluation and Research, "We see the need to get the concept across that this is for keeps. You can be sloppy when you are dealing with a scientific paper, but you can't be sloppy when you are dealing with a human."[24]

Experimental Phases

Meanwhile, other researchers are looking closely at the vectors—the viruses that have long been used as the Trojan horses to deliver the new genes to a patient's cells. While safer viruses have been found and employed since the death of Jesse Gelsinger, some scientists wonder whether viruses need to be used at all. At Case Western Reserve University in Cleveland, Ohio, researchers have experimented with injecting the genes into liposomes—globules of fat—that are tiny enough to pass through the cellular walls. After the liposome enters the cell, it spits out a peptide—a portion of a protein molecule—that carries the new gene into the cell nucleus. At Case Western Reserve, physicians have injected liposomes carrying healthy genes into mice. Tests revealed that the liposomes successfully delivered the genes without causing the animals' immune systems to react.

Although research into the use of liposomes as the Trojan horse continues, many scientists harbor doubts about the eventual success of the therapy. Unlike viruses, liposomes do not seek out cells to infect; they move passively through the blood. Therefore, many liposomes will likely bypass the targets. Far fewer cells will receive the new DNA, which could reduce the likelihood that the therapy will be successful. Also, some researchers have reported that after the liposome has entered the cell, it does not always spit out the peptide.

liposomes

Globules of fat that are able to penetrate cell walls to deliver DNA; they are not as effective as viruses because they move passively through the blood and do not seek out cells to infect.

Other scientists are studying the use of bacteria as a Trojan horse. As with viruses, bacteria can spread disease. However, most bacteria respond to antibiotic drugs like penicillin or amoxicillin. Therefore, scientists are looking at the possibility of inserting new genes into bacteria, then injecting the bacteria into the patient. If the patient develops an immune reaction to the bacteria, a physician would quickly inject the patient with an antibiotic drug. Swiss genetics researcher Guido Dietrich points out that bacteria have long been used to fashion vaccines against such diseases as tuberculosis and typhoid fever, so it has already been proven safe to use bacteria to treat diseases. "There should be no safety issue,"[25] he says.

At Purdue University in Indiana, researchers have used *Listeria monocytogenes* bacteria to deliver genes to mice. The bacteria cause the disease listeriosis, which manifests itself in fever, nausea, and diarrhea and typically lasts for about two weeks. First, the Purdue researchers added human genes to *Listeria monocytogenes* bacteria, then injected the bacteria into human cells they had cultured in a lab dish. The human cells were then injected into mice. An analysis of blood drawn from the mice indicated that about 40 percent of the human cells were penetrated by the DNA-carrying bacteria.

Clearly, the use of bacteria as well as liposomes are still in highly experimental phases, and, at least for now, the Trojan horses that are used to deliver the genes to the patients will be launched in the form of viruses. Certainly, scientists as well as government regulators are much more on guard now than they were a decade ago when Jesse Gelsinger received a massive dose of a virus that sparked the immune reaction that killed him. Still, there is no denying the dangers of introducing a potentially harmful virus into the body of a patient who is already ill.

Attacking Bad Genes with Drugs

Although gene replacement therapy remains an experimental process, available to perhaps only a few hundred patients a year participating in clinical trials, the study of genes has nevertheless provided assistance to medicine for several decades. The secrets unearthed by Watson, Crick, and the other pioneers of the science have helped improve the lives of many thousands of people. Mostly, genetic science has provided applications toward the production of new medications. For example, since 1982 drug companies have been able to manufacture insulin using genetically altered bacteria. People who suffer from diabetes are unable to make insulin naturally and, therefore, often need daily injections of the chemical in order for their bodies to metabolize sugar, turning it into energy. To make the chemical, drug makers insert insulin-producing human genes into *E. coli* bacteria, which are used because they grow and divide quickly, enhancing the production of insulin.

When specific genes are identified as disease triggers, medications can be designed to turn off the culprit genes to block their effects or turn on other genes to neutralize the bad genes. "We should be very clear on this point," says British genetics researcher Walter Bodmer, "The future of development of new pharmaceuticals in the 21st century will rest squarely with the mapping and sequencing of our genes. With the identification of the triggers . . . we should be able to develop drugs that will block them so halting the pernicious progress of diseases, for instance in conditions such as Alzheimer's disease."[26]

Turning Off the Alzheimer's Gene

Alzheimer's disease was first diagnosed a century ago by German physician Alois Alzheimer. Patients develop a plaque on their brain cells that robs them of their memories. The disease is progressive—most Alzheimer's patients start out by forgetting little things: the day of the week or the names of close friends and relatives. In time, Alzheimer's patients essentially find themselves living in a fog of dementia, unable to dress or feed themselves, completely oblivious to the world around them. More than 5 million Americans, most of them elderly, suffer from Alzheimer's disease.

There is no question that Alzheimer's is an inherited disease—scientists believe the gene identified as HDAC2 is responsible for creating enzymes that cause the plaque buildup on cells. The development of medications that turn off the HDAC2 gene may be the best hope for Alzheimer's disease patients. Scientists at the Massachusetts Institute of Technology (MIT) have announced the preliminary results of a drug that inhibits the release of the plaque-causing enzymes. So far, the researchers have experimented only on mice. To perform the test, the scientists injected a gene into the mice to induce Alzheimer's symptoms, then charted the reduction of the rodents' mental abilities. When it appeared that the mice were exhibiting symptoms similar to Alzheimer's disease, the animals were injected with the test drug. After a short period of time, the mice regained their memories and even learned new tasks.

The results of the drug trials on mice were announced in 2009; scientists believe human trials are not likely to commence for several years. Still, advocates for people with Alzheimer's disease see the development of medications that can turn on or turn off genes as the best hope for patients. "We need to do more research to investigate whether developing treatments that control this gene could benefit people with Alzheimer's,"[27] says Rebecca Wood, executive director of the Alzheimer's Research Trust, a patient advocacy group in Great Britain.

> ## smart drugs
>
> Class of drugs designed to head straight for the genes causing the illnesses; unlike radiation and chemotherapy, the drugs target the malignant cells only, leaving healthy cells alone.

Curing Cystic Fibrosis

One drug undergoing clinical trials on human patients is aimed at wiping out cystic fibrosis, which afflicts some 30,000 Americans a year. Ten million Americans are believed to carry the gene that causes cystic fibrosis, meaning they can pass it on to their children who can also pass it on, ensuring that the disease will remain part of human biology for generations to come. Cystic fibrosis produces excessive amounts of mucus in the lungs and other organs, often proving fatal to patients by the time they reach their thirties. The faulty gene fails to produce a protein that

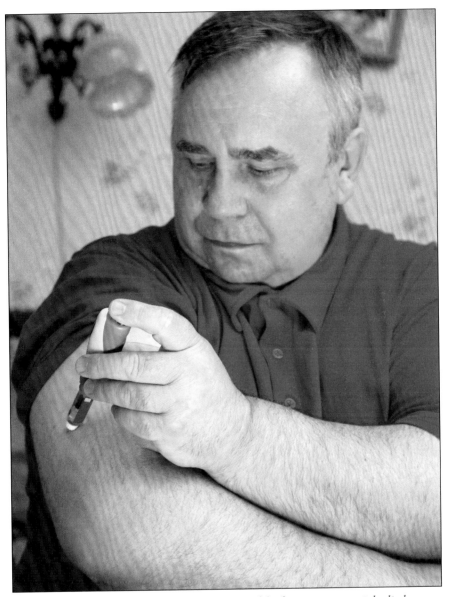

A daily injection of insulin makes it possible for a person with diabetes to metabolize sugar, which provides the body with energy. Drug-making companies have used genetically altered bacteria to produce large quantities of insulin.

helps the body cleanse its cells of chloride. It is the overabundance of chloride in cells that causes the mucus buildup in the organs.

Chrissy Falletti was diagnosed with cystic fibrosis six weeks after her birth in 1975. Since then, the Ohio schoolteacher has had to endure not only the disease but the therapies that have enabled her to function.

⚛ What Is Xenotransplantation?

If genetically altered milk from animals can be used to develop drugs for humans, could whole organs from animals be genetically altered to replace human organs? Many scientists believe it is possible.

Many transplant patients find themselves on waiting lists for human organs. According to the United Network for Organ Sharing, the non-profit organization that matches donor organs with recipients, 80,000 Americans are on waiting lists for new kidneys, hearts, and other organs. Because of the scarcity of donors, 5,000 people die each year while waiting for organs to become available.

Doctors have experimented with xenotransplantation—the use of animal organs in place of human organs—but the transplants have met with failure because of the human body's tendency to reject the animal organs. Some gene therapists believe that by genetically altering animals, their organs may become useful for transplantation. The key is to eliminate the animals' genes that trigger the rejection of their organs by the human body's immune system. Researchers have already announced their success in removing the trigger gene in pigs, labeled GGTA1.

While it may be decades before whole organs from animals can be transplanted into humans, doctors believe they can transplant genetically altered pig cells known as islets, which produce insulin, into the pancreases of human diabetes patients. The pancreas is the organ that manufactures insulin. In 2006 doctors at the University of Minnesota transplanted pig islets into the pancreases of diabetic monkeys, which were able to survive without insulin injections for the duration of the 100-day trial. Meanwhile, gene therapy researchers in Russia, Mexico, and New Zealand have reported they have already transplanted pig islets into human diabetes patients.

Each day she consumes 15 medications that help control the buildup of mucus in her body. Moreover, twice a day she must wear a contraption that resembles a life vest: Hoses inflate the vest, providing pressure on her chest that breaks up the mucus. At night, her husband must clap her on the back, the sides, and chest to break up the mucus before bed. "It takes about three hours out of my day to clear my airway,"[28] she says. Even those precautions have not always kept Falletti healthy—she has suffered numerous bouts of pneumonia and nearly died due to lung failure. She also struggles to keep weight on. Now in her mid-thirties, Falletti has arrived at the age when many cystic fibrosis patients die.

In the case of cystic fibrosis, gene replacement therapy has not shown promising results; after the cystic fibrosis gene was identified in 1989, researchers attempted to replace it with healthy genes. Experiments worked in the test tube, but human patients rejected the viruses that delivered the healthy genes. Instead, researchers have turned in a different direction, concentrating on a medication to help the body produce the chloride-cleansing protein that the faulty gene fails to produce. Therefore, in this case gene replacement therapy was not used to treat cystic fibrosis, but by identifying the gene that sparks cystic fibrosis, drug companies believe they can tailor medications to perform the tasks the faulty genes are unable to do. In this case the drug produces the protein that cleanses chloride from the cells of patients. Falletti participated in the human trials of the drug, produced by Vertex Pharmaceuticals of Cambridge, Massachusetts. After four weeks on the drug, Falletti's lung function improved by nearly 20 percent. Moreover, as a cystic fibrosis patient she coughed hundreds of times a day, but while taking the experimental drug her fits of coughing virtually disappeared. She also gained weight. Finally, though, the drug trial ended, and Falletti was forced to give up the experimental medication. Now, she is eagerly awaiting the public release of the medication as the drug goes through further trials and the FDA decides whether it is safe to make available for widespread consumption. She says, "When you've finally felt what normal feels like, you kind of realize it's not that much fun being your abnormal self."[29]

Development of Smart Drugs

The pursuit of drugs to treat some cancers has also benefited from the study of genes. By identifying genes in cancer cells, doctors have been able to tell which drugs are more effective in fighting those cells. For example, physicians have identified a specific gene, which has been labeled HER2, as responsible for causing about 25 percent of breast cancer cases. The real culprit is the protein produced by the HER2 gene. That protein sits atop cells in the breast, controlling their growth and division. When there is an abundance of the HER2 protein, cells often turn cancerous and also grow and divide at an accelerated rate.

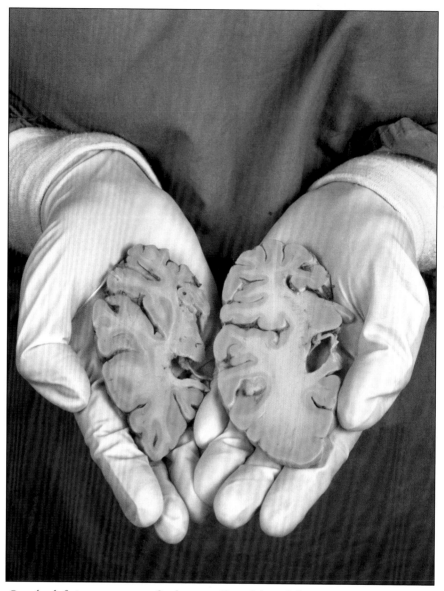

On the left is a segment of a brain affected by Alzheimer's disease; on the right is a segment of a healthy brain. Researchers have identified a gene that may cause Alzheimer's disease. They are working on medications that will turn off the gene.

In 1998 the California drug company Genentech Inc. received permission from the FDA to market a drug specifically designed to attack the HER2 protein. The drug, Herceptin, attaches itself to the HER2 protein and summons antibodies to attack the cancerous cells. Moreover, Herceptin has also been found to slow the growth and division of the cancerous cells. Louise Cooper was among the first patients to be treated with Herceptin. That was in 1998. The drug cured her cancer, and now Cooper has made the most of her second chance at life—she has climbed mountains on 4 continents and has made plans to visit Antarctica. "I feel blessed," said Cooper, 55. "How can you complain when you were supposed to die?"[30]

Many doctors urge their patients to use Herceptin in concert with chemotherapy, which is a common treatment for cancer that includes ingesting drugs that attack not only the cancerous cells but healthy cells as well. Many chemotherapy patients grow ill from the treatments and must endure long periods of nausea, fatigue, hair loss, pain, and other symptoms. Doctors equate chemotherapy to the military tactic of "carpet bombing," a style of assault that wipes out everything and everyone in the target zone, whether they are enemy combatants or innocent civilians.

The next step in genetic-based drug therapy is to find drugs that are so effective that chemotherapy may no longer be necessary. These

> **pharmacogenomics**
>
> The study of how genes react to drugs.

are known as smart drugs because they go directly to the gene that is triggering the cancer. "I can't imagine a kinder or gentler way of killing cancer cells without injuring the patient," says George Demetri, a physician at Dana-Farber Cancer Institute in Boston, Massachusetts. "Why kill normal cells and hope that you happen to have a lot of cancer cells in your field of treatment? Why pummel the patient with toxic chemotherapy? Why not just give a drug that helps the body get rid of mutated cells?"[31]

One Size Fits All

Smart drugs would not only be a step forward for cancer patients but for anybody who takes prescription drugs. Indeed, it is estimated that half of all drugs prescribed in America have no positive effect on the people taking them. That is because a drug is typically formulated in a "one size fits all" protocol that does not take into account the genetic differences from patient to patient.

A typical case involved Jody Uslan, a 52-year-old Los Angeles, California, woman who was treated for breast cancer. After the cancer was wiped out using conventional methods, Uslan took regular doses of tamoxifen, a drug designed to prevent a reoccurrence of breast tumors. After two years on tamoxifen, Uslan took a genetic test that revealed the drug was not effective and that she was still in danger of developing new tumors. "I was devastated," she said. "You find out you've been taking this medication for all of this time, and then you find you are not getting any benefit."[32]

In Uslan's case, tamoxifen did not work. In most cases an enzyme in the body, known as CYP2DG, converts the drug into the chemical endoxifen, which is a cancer-fighting agent. But the genetic test revealed Uslan's body lacks CYP2DG—as do 7 percent of all people. In fact, a 2005 study revealed that 32 percent of breast cancer patients whose bodies lack CYP2DG suffer relapses within 2 years of their treatments to eradicate their tumors. Currently, no known drug therapies are available to these women.

Still, the drive to end the "one size fits all" protocol in drug development has spawned a new science known as pharmacogenomics—the study of how genes react to drugs. Pharmacogenomics looks at whether drug makers can tinker with the chemistry of the drugs so that they will more closely fit the genetic properties of the individual patients. Essentially, drug makers are being asked to personalize their drugs. Of course, patients would then have to be tested to find out whether they are a good fit for the drugs. Some drugs have already undergone such testing—according to the FDA, about 200 prescription drugs already on the market have been identified as being most effective only for patients who are a good genetic match for the drugs.

It is a branch of science and medicine that could potentially revolutionize drug therapies. Nevertheless, the creation of new drugs tailored to the genetic makeup of individual patients is years if not decades in the future. Indeed, after pharmacogenomics researchers start producing drugs, 10 years or more may go by before the FDA grants approval for their use. Typically, new drugs must go through extensive clinical trial periods and be proven safe before the federal government approves their distribution to the public. People who are pursuing pharmacogenomics inside the drug industry are well aware that they are developing new ways of making drugs, and even they are not sure how the process will turn out. "There are lots of biomarkers in use now that have never been through stringent trials," says Donna Mendrick, a researcher for Gene Logic, a Maryland company that provides genetic analyses. "We in industry are setting up a process that was never used before."[33]

Three More Years of Life

One of the first drugs developed specifically to attack a faulty gene is Gleevec, which is manufactured by the Swiss drug company Novartis. Gleevec received FDA approval in 2001. The drug is used to treat patients who suffer from stomach cancer. The condition is caused by a

 Gene Doping

In 2006 German track coach Thomas Springstein was tried on charges of furnishing performance-enhancing drugs to young athletes. Such charges are not unusual; many such cases have been reported in the United States. In Springstein's case, the drug he was charged with giving to athletes was Repoxygen, a medication that is ordinarily used to treat anemia. People who have anemia are deficient in red blood cells, which causes them to suffer from weakness and chronic fatigue. (Springstein was convicted and received a suspended sentence of 16 months, which means he did not have to spend time in jail.)

Repoxygen is a gene therapy drug—it works by delivering a human gene to a patient's cells, prompting the cells to manufacture a hormone which, in turn, drives the production of red blood cells. In healthy people, Repoxygen would theoretically provide an extra boost of energy—which would explain why track athletes might be willing to try the drug.

The case has alarmed sports officials throughout the world who fear that "gene doping" may become more common once gene therapies become more widespread. Instead of taking performance-enhancing drugs, officials fear, athletes will find ways to be injected with genes that could help them become faster and stronger. "It doesn't matter how weird and wacky it sounds, playing around with genes is about as out-there as anything I've ever heard of," says Boulder, Colorado, track coach Darren De Reuck, who has helped train Olympic athletes. "I'm sure some people will think it would be a great thing to try."

Quoted in Gretchen Reynolds, "Outlaw DNA," *New York Times*, June 3, 2007. www.nytimes.com.

faulty gene that produces a protein which prompts cells to turn cancerous, growing and dividing at a tremendous pace. Gleevec stymies the function of the protein and also kills the cancerous cells. Despite its promise, in many patients the drug has proven to be just a temporary treatment.

First diagnosed with stomach cancer in 1999, Ken Garabadian of Massachusetts was facing a bleak future. In many cancer patients, doctors can cut out the tumors and kill remaining malignant cells through chemotherapy or radiation treatments, in which cancerous cells are killed by radioactive beams. (And, like chemotherapy, radiation therapy often causes severe side effects, including nausea, fatigue, and hair loss.) In Garabadian's case, though, his tumor had already ruptured, spreading cancerous cells over a widespread area of his digestive tract. New tumors had formed. Surgery was no longer an option; his cancer was regarded as incurable.

Garabadian started taking Gleevec in 2002, and the drug soon showed amazing results: His tumors started dying on the first day of treatment and completely disappeared within weeks. "This was the first time in the United States that any solid tumor had ever been stopped in its tracks with no major side effects after a relatively short period of treatment," said David G. Nathan, the former head of Dana-Farber Cancer Institute, where Garabadian was treated. "The tumors shrank and remained invisible in Ken's abdomen . . . Ken became a poster boy for advanced cancer clinical and basic research. He spoke widely about the importance of optimism and determination in dealing with cancer and for being on the cutting edge of cancer research."[34]

transgenic animals

Animals that have been genetically altered by insertion of human genes into their chromosomes.

The patient was able to stay cancer-free for three years, but eventually the tumors returned. His doctors believe that Garabadian's body built up a resistance to Gleevec and, eventually, the drug lost its ability to stop the cancerous protein. That type of reaction is common in cancer patients—cancer cells are notoriously able to adapt to their environments, and therefore, after only three years of treatment, the cancer cells in Garabadian's body mutated again, rendering Gleevec impotent. He died in 2005. Nevertheless, a drug produced through genetic research

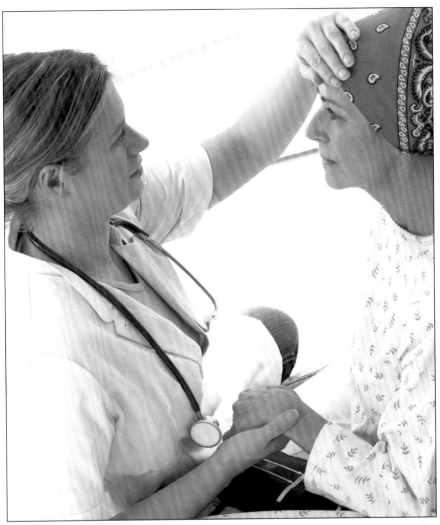

Chemotherapy, which is the most common treatment for cancer, typically results in long bouts of nausea, fatigue, hair loss, and pain. Genetic-based drug therapy may lead to the development of alternatives to harsh treatments such as chemotherapy.

managed to extend Garabadian's life by three years, giving doctors hope that in time, better and smarter drugs can be developed that will further extend the lives of cancer patients.

Animal Pharming

Some smart drugs are being developed by tinkering with genes found in animals—this technique is known as animal pharming. It requires the use of transgenic animals—animals that have been genetically altered by insertion of human genes into their chromosomes. The animals then produce a protein in their milk, urine, blood, sperm, or eggs that can be employed in medications for human diseases.

Scientists see many advantages in using animals as bioreactors, which are living organisms that naturally produce proteins or other chemicals that can be used in drugs. For starters, culturing cells in a laboratory to produce the proteins needed for drugs is expensive and labor-intensive—the cultures must constantly be monitored by scientists and technicians while they grow. Moreover, it takes a lot of expensive lab machinery to grow the cultures using artificial techniques. Finally, isolating and purifying the proteins is a highly specialized process that is often incredibly difficult to accomplish in a test tube. Typically, labs that culture proteins for gene therapy run on budgets of tens of millions of dollars a year.

Why not just inject the genes into a cow and let the cow culture the protein naturally? According to the FDA, it costs between $20,000 and $300,000 to nurture and maintain a transgenic animal, but that animal is capable of producing, in its lifetime, pharmaceuticals valued at between $200 million and $300 million.

In 1999 the first farm dedicated to raising animals specifically for pharmaceutical purposes was established in Vienna, Wisconsin. The farm is owned by a Netherlands company, Pharming Group, which operates pharmaceutical production companies in a number of countries. The farm started with 13 calves that were injected with human genes. Since then, the farm's herd has increased to some 200 head of genetically altered cows whose milk has been used to culture proteins for human medicine.

bioreactors

Living organisms that naturally produce proteins or other chemicals that can be employed in the development of drugs.

By 2009 Pharming Group was reported to have two major drugs in development. One of those drugs is Rhucin, a medication designed to control hereditary angioedema, an inherited disease that causes swelling, hoarseness, and abdominal cramping. The disease is caused by the lack of a protein known as C1 in the cells of patients. The other drug is Prodarsan, which is designed to treat patients who suffer from a rare disease known as Cockayne syndrome. Patients with this inherited disease suffer from sensitivity to sunlight, premature aging, hearing loss, blindness, and impaired development of their central nervous systems. The proteins from two faulty genes, identified as ERCC6 and ERCC8, have been identified as the causes of Cockayne syndrome.

Medications Offer Hope for the Future

As with most new drugs, the widespread release of medications developed through animal pharming is likely to be years in the future. Drugs designed to attack faulty genes, whether they are synthesized in a laboratory or cultured in the bodies of cows, are among the most advanced form of drugs in development. That is why most of them are still being tested on laboratory animals. And yet, if they produce the type of results in humans that they are showing in mice, it is likely that these drugs will eventually have a major impact on cancer, cystic fibrosis, Alzheimer's disease, and other horrific illnesses that cost millions of human lives every year.

Stem Cells, Cloning, and Gene Therapy

L ike Ashanthi DeSilva, Katlyn Demerchant suffered from bubble boy disease. But Katlyn's case was much more severe: While Ashanthi had been able to live at home with her family, Katlyn spent the first 15 months of her life in a completely sterile hospital environment near her family's home in New Brunswick, Canada. To visit Katlyn, her parents wore sterile gowns, gloves, germ-proof masks, and protective booties on their shoes and were urged by doctors not to pick up their baby. Even under these conditions, doctors had given the Demerchants a grim prognosis for their daughter: Unless cured of the condition, it was likely she would die at a young age.

Eventually, Katlyn's case came to the attention of doctors at the NIH in Bethesda—the same lab that had treated Ashanthi. In May 2007 Katlyn arrived at the NIH lab to begin gene therapy.

Receiving New Genes Through Stem Cells

In Katlyn's case, the doctors elected to try a different therapy than had been administered to Ashanthi. First, healthy genes were injected into a virus, but instead of injecting the vector directly into the child, the doctors withdrew stem cells from Katlyn's bone marrow. These cells were exposed to the virus and then injected back into Katlyn's bone marrow.

Found in the body, stem cells are undifferentiated, meaning they have not yet become cells of the liver, or of the blood, or of any other part of the body. In stem cell therapy, doctors coax the undifferentiated cells into replacing cells that are damaged or diseased.

Soon after the undifferentiated stem cells were returned to Katlyn's body, they started taking on characteristics of bone marrow cells. Now, the new bone marrow cells included the healthy genes that were able to spark the proteins providing Katlyn's immunity to infection. Following the therapy, Katlyn returned to the New Brunswick hospital, but five months later tests confirmed that the child's blood was now manufacturing antibodies that ensured her immunity against disease. On that day,

Katlyn's parents took their toddler outside the hospital for her first walk in the sunshine. "She started running around and asking us a million questions," said her mother, Daisy Demerchant. "She'd point to the sun, clouds, leaves, cars, everything imaginable, and ask us what it was. Ever since that day, she has never wanted to stay inside."[35] A few months after their daughter received her new genes, the Demerchants took her home.

Stem cell therapy is a separate branch of medical science that is believed to have widespread potential for curing many diseases. These include Parkinson's disease, a neurological disorder that manifests itself in slowed and slurred speech, muscle tremors, and rigid muscles; as well as Alzheimer's disease, some cancers, and amyotrophic lateral sclerosis, also known as Lou Gehrig's disease, which is a devastating disease of the brain and central nervous system. In addition, people who have been paralyzed in accidents may regain use of their limbs because, it is believed, stem cells can be coaxed into becoming new cells that can rebuild damaged tissue in the spinal cord.

> **undifferentiated**
>
> Status of stem cells before they form into specific, or differentiated, tissues or fluids in the body; scientists can coax stem cells into replacing diseased cells.

Like gene therapy, stem cell therapy is still very much in an experimental phase—most patients receiving stem cell treatments are part of clinical trials. Nevertheless, Katlyn's case represents a step in moving both therapies forward, showing the enormous potential of what can be accomplished by combining these two cutting-edge branches of medical science.

Stem Cell Research Progresses

The foundation for modern-day stem cell research was laid in the late nineteenth century and early twentieth century, when scientists discovered the ability of some animals to regrow parts of their bodies that had been injured (or intentionally lopped off in the laboratory.) For the most part, these were simple animals such as flatworms, newts, and zebra fish. It soon became evident that the animals were employing stem cells to regenerate new tissue. In 1895 a German zoologist, Valentin Häcker, first used the term *Stammzelle*—in English, "stem cell"—to describe undifferentiated cells he withdrew from a crustacean known as a cyclops, a tiny sea animal similar to a lobster.

Häcker found the cyclops stem cells in a blastocyst, which is an embryo that is no more than a few days old. In humans, the blastocyst forms

Fear of Eugenics

If reproductive cloning is pursued, some critics worry that eugenics may not be far behind. The concept of eugenics suggests the weak and ill should be eliminated from the species, which would grow stronger if it does not have to contend with genetically caused diseases or debilitations.

Eugenics was conceived by Francis Galton, a cousin of Charles Darwin, in an 1869 book titled *Hereditary Genius*. Galton suggested that eugenics would be the next logical step following Darwin's theory of natural selection. That theory holds that over time—in most cases, tens of thousands of years—species of plants and animals improve because they evolve using the best traits provided by their ancestors. In Galton's view, humans could give natural selection a bit of a shove.

Galton believed if mentally disabled people were not allowed to produce children, eventually there would be no mentally disabled people—certainly, no mentally disabled people whose intellectual capabilities failed to develop because of flaws in their genes. The end result, Galton believed, would be that the human race would improve.

Galton's ideas gained the support of some of the leading intellectuals of the era, including authors H.G. Wells, Émile Zola, and George Bernard Shaw. Even among the proponents of eugenics, though, it appears that some believed the theory was flawed. The beautiful dancer Isadora Duncan is said to have once proposed marriage to Shaw, suggesting that their child would be both brilliant and beautiful. The gaunt and balding Shaw replied, "But what, my dear, if the poor thing should have my body and your brain?"

Quoted in Dave Kindred, "A Cryonic Shame," *Sporting News*, July 29, 2002, p. 64.

about five days after conception; it includes about 150 to 200 cells and is no larger than a grain of sand. These cells are regarded as "pluripotent," meaning they have the potential to develop into almost any kind of cell in any part of the body.

These stem cells are known as embryonic stem cells because they are withdrawn from embryos. To obtain the embryos for stem cell research, scientists use blastocysts that are donated by in vitro fertilization clinics. These are clinics that help infertile couples conceive. At the clinics, eggs are surgically removed from the woman and fertilized in a lab dish with sperm provided by the man. After fertilization, the egg is returned to the woman's womb. To ensure the success of the procedure, clinic doctors typically withdraw and fertilize several eggs, but only one egg is returned to the womb. The other embryos are frozen and eventually discarded, but many couples agree to donate the embryos to stem cell research labs.

Because of its potential for eradicating disease, stem cell research has widespread support among Americans as well as political leaders. A 2008 poll by *Time* magazine showed 73 percent of Americans favoring the use of embryos for stem cell research, but advancements in the science slowed between 2001 and 2009 when President George W. Bush refused to provide billions of dollars in federal aid to laboratories pursuing embryonic stem cell research. Bush and other conservative political leaders said they could not support the destruction of human life, regardless of how early its stage of development may be.

Twice during Bush's presidency Congress attempted to overturn Bush's ban on funding for embryonic stem cell research, but the efforts by Congress fell short. Members of the House and Senate were unable to muster enough votes to override Bush's vetoes. In 2009, just three months after taking office, President Barack Obama signed an executive order clearing the way for federal funds to be used for stem cell research.

> **blastocyst**
>
> A very young embryo, no more than five days old. The blastocyst contains about 150 to 200 stem cells.

Combining Gene Therapy and Stem Cell Therapy

During the Bush presidency embryonic stem cell research may have been slowed, but the research, supported with private funds, did not stop. Hundreds of stem cell research programs were carried out at private and university labs, and some of them looked very hard at combining gene therapy with stem cell therapy. The concept calls for the addition of new DNA to the stem cells so that when they are injected into the patient's body, they will differentiate into healthy cells that will contain copies of healthy genes, replacing genes in the body that are defective. "Instead of gene therapy being done in the patient, as is the case in cancer, it's being done in the cells in a laboratory before doctors use them for therapy,"[36] says Ronald G. Crystal, chief of pulmonary care at Weill Cornell Medical Center in New York City.

Stem cells can be drawn from blastocysts, but there is also a second source for the cells—the patients themselves. Scientists have found that stem cells can also be found in bone marrow, brain matter, skin, intestines, teeth, internal organs, and other places in the body. These are known as adult stem cells. Their use is much less controversial because the therapy does not require destruction of human embryos.

Gene therapy employing adult stem cells has already shown results—Katlyn's stem cells were withdrawn from her bone marrow. Bone marrow also provided stem cells for a 2009 trial conducted jointly by the Salk Institute and the Center for Regenerative Medicine in Barcelona, Spain, in which scientists took steps toward treating an inherited disorder known as Fanconi anemia, or FA.

FA is a rare disorder that results in stunted growth and bone deformities; the disease often progresses into leukemia. FA has been traced to malfunctions in 13 genes. As part of the experiment, the scientists withdrew bone marrow stem cells from FA patients, then injected the cells with viruses containing healthy genes. The experiment ended there. The scientists did not inject the genetically altered stem cells back into the patients; they simply wanted to see how the stem cells reacted to the introduction of the viruses and the new genes. They acknowledged that the therapy is too new and untested to risk the lives of the patients. "In the future it may become possible to transfer the corrected stem cells back into the patient, but much work needs to be done before this can be transferred from the lab bench to the bedside,"[37] said Chris Matthew, a molecular geneticist who has pursued similar research at King's College in London.

Altering the Embryo

While some scientists attempt to genetically alter stem cells, others are pursuing a therapy that would alter the embryo so that it would produce genetically correct stem cells. These stem cells would then be used to treat diseases and debilitations in patients. This process is known as somatic cell nuclear transfer (SCNT). Another name for the science is therapeutic cloning.

In SCNT, a nucleus is withdrawn from a human somatic cell, which is a cell that contains genetic information from both parents and therefore a complete set of the patient's DNA. The nucleus is then inserted into an unfertilized egg that has had its nucleus removed. The process essentially transfers a complete set of genetic information from the somatic

Devastating Brain Diseases

Parkinson's and Alzheimer's are degenerative brain diseases. Although scientists do not know what causes either disease, they have a good understanding of what takes place in the brains of people who suffer from them. Gene therapy and stem cell therapy, or the two combined, offer great promise for treating diseases such as these in the future.

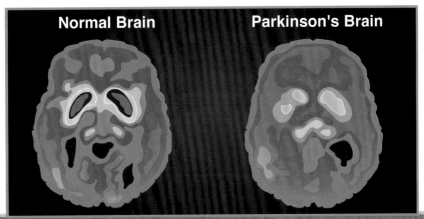

Parkinson's occurs due to the gradual loss of nerve cells in particular areas of the brain. This halts the production of dopamine, a brain chemical that is essential for proper functioning of the nervous system and smooth, coordinated muscle movement. The above illustrations show the difference between a normal brain (left) and the brain of a Parkinson's patient (right).

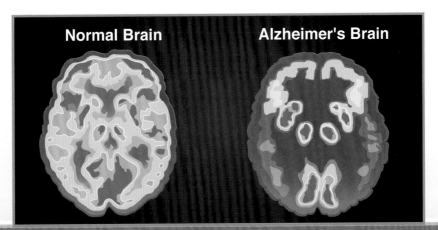

Alzheimer's is a fatal disease that is characterized by an abnormal buildup of proteins in the brain called plaques and tangles, which cause the brain to waste away over time. The above illustrations show the difference between a brain with normal activity (left) and a brain that has been atrophied because of Alzheimer's (right).

Sources: The National Academies, "Understanding Stem Cells," October 2006. http://dels.nas.edu; National Institute on Aging, "The Changing Brain in Alzheimer's Disease," August 29, 2006. www.nia.nih.gov.

cell into an egg. After being infused with the nucleus from the somatic cell, the egg starts to divide, similar to how it would divide after naturally being penetrated by a sperm. After a few days, stem cells will form that are genetically identical to the donor of the somatic cell. Doctors will then inject the stem cells into the patient, where they replace damaged cells in the spinal cord, brain, or other organs.

Many researchers believe therapeutic cloning can provide the most effective and safest form of gene therapy. Unlike other forms of gene therapy, the stem cells are usually not delivered in a virus and would pose no danger to the bodies of recipients. Also, stem cells have the ability to self-renew, meaning there is no need to constantly replace the faulty genes with healthy genes, because the stem cells make the healthy genetic material on their own. As with other forms of gene therapy, though, therapeutic cloning remains a highly experimental process that so far has been confined to the laboratory and limited trials on humans.

Concerns About Cloning

Therapeutic cloning has sparked opposition from many critics because they fear the science could also be used for reproductive cloning. In other words, if it is possible to genetically engineer a human embryo so that it can provide stem cells to fight cancer or repair a shattered spinal cord, is it also possible to genetically engineer a human embryo to ensure the baby is born with blue eyes, an athletic physique, or movie idol looks? "Offensive, grotesque, revolting, repugnant and repulsive—those are the words most commonly heard regarding the prospect of human cloning," says Leon R. Kass, an adjunct professor at the Washington, D.C.–based conservative think tank, the American Enterprise Institute.

Such reactions come from both the man or woman on the street and from the intellectuals, the believers and atheists, humanists and scientists. . . . People are repelled by many aspects of human cloning. They recoil from the prospect of mass production of human beings, with large clones of look-alikes, compromised in their individuality; the idea of father-son or mother-daughter twins, the bizarre prospects of a woman's giving birth to and rearing a genetic copy of herself, her spouse, or even her deceased father or mother; the grotesqueness of conceiving a child as an exact replacement for another who has died. [38]

Reproductive cloning involves the insertion of DNA into an egg. Unlike therapeutic cloning, in reproductive cloning the egg is then placed back in the womb of the mother where the embryo develops into a fetus and then grows naturally. Eventually, the child is born as though he or she were conceived through the sexual act.

Reproductive cloning has already been performed on animals—it was most famously accomplished in 1996 by doctors in Scotland who cloned a sheep named Dolly. It took the scientists 276 tries before

Gene Therapy Improves Chemotherapy

Because chemotherapy causes many side effects, including nausea, anemia, bleeding, and fatigue, doctors often scale back the doses they provide to cancer patients. Using gene therapy and stem cells, doctors at the Ireland Cancer Center in Cleveland, Ohio, believe they can make cancer patients tolerate the chemotherapy better, which means they can receive stronger doses of the tumor-killing drugs.

Doctors withdrew stem cells from the bone marrow of six cancer patients, then added a gene identified as MGMT to the cells. The stem cells carrying the new gene were then returned to the patients.

During prior tests on lab animals, MGMT was found to help mice build up resistance to chemotherapy drugs, enabling the animals to endure higher doses. The new genes also helped the human patients endure higher doses of chemotherapy. Twenty-eight weeks after injection of the new genes, the patients continued to show strong resistance to the noxious drugs. "This study is the first to show the success of treatment with evidence that stem cells now carry the new gene," said Stanton Gerson, the cancer specialist who headed the study. "These patients show the success of treatment with evidence that their stem cells now carry the new genes. This is a breakthrough."

Quoted in *Science Daily*, "Advancing Stem Cell Gene Therapy," December 16, 2007. www.sciencedaily.com.

Embryonic stem cells, visible in this color-enhanced scanning electron micrograph, are able to differentiate into any of the 200 cell types in the human body. The combining of gene therapy with stem cell therapy offers enormous promise.

they successfully transferred another sheep's DNA into the egg that produced Dolly.

Now more than a decade later, reproductive cloning continues to be a highly experimental process with just a few dozen animals—mice, cats, pigs, horses, and dogs—known to have been born through the cloning process. "We are still surprised that cloning works,"[39] says Ian Wilmut, the Scottish scientist who led the team that created Dolly. In fact, less than 5 percent of the eggs injected with DNA result in live births. Moreover, although Dolly seemed to be healthy—she later gave birth to five lambs—she died at the age of six, meaning she lived about half as long as sheep are expected to live.

> ## therapeutic cloning
>
> Officially known as somatic cell nuclear transfer, therapeutic cloning is the technique of introducing new DNA into an egg whose own DNA has been removed.

Animal cloning is pursued because cloned animals, like pharmed animals, can help manufacture genes that can become components of human medications. Also, cloning animals can ensure that no species would ever become extinct. As long as an animal's DNA has been preserved, the species can be maintained despite environmental changes, diseases, hunting, and other factors that drive species into extinction.

Although there have been cloning experiments on human embryos, due to strict federal laws no embryos have been permitted to mature beyond the blastocyst stage. Still, bioethicists and others worry that reproductive cloning can be pursued in other countries where governments do not keep close watch over medical research.

The Strange Saga of Ted Williams

While the prospect that humans could be cloned and churned out as though they were produced in a factory is offensive to many people, the financial gains that could be realized through the science may be too lucrative for some to resist. Soon after baseball legend Ted Williams

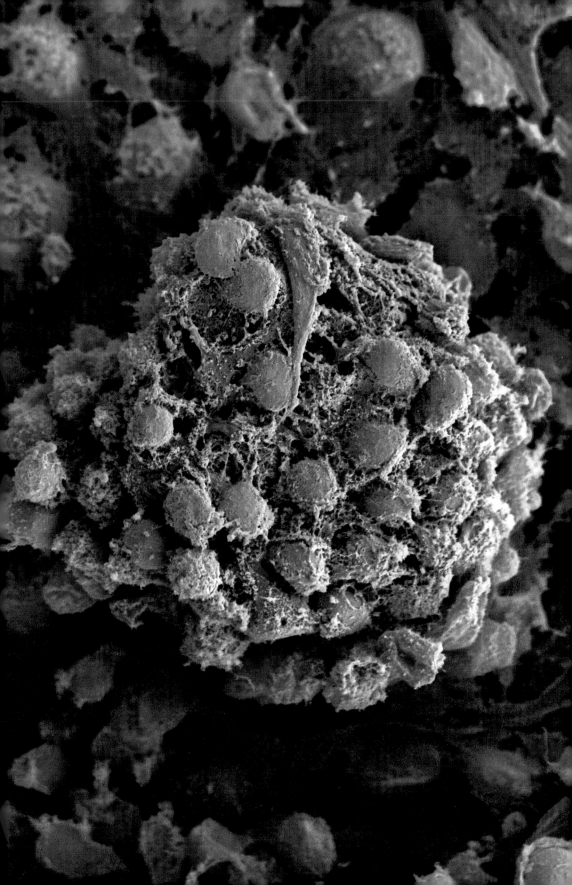

died in 2002, a bizarre story was broken by reporters at *Sports Illustrated*. Williams's son John Henry had the body of his father frozen in liquid nitrogen, and some members of the Williams family were charging that John Henry intended to eventually sell his father's DNA to parents who desired to splice the slugger's genes into the chromosomes of their offspring so they, too, would grow up to be all-star major leaguers. John Henry is alleged to have told his sister, "Wouldn't it be neat to sell Dad's DNA? There are lots of people who would pay big bucks to have little Ted Williamses running around."[40]

reproductive cloning

A technique in which an embryo is genetically engineered to ensure the offspring is born with certain characteristics.

The notion of cloning Ted Williams could certainly find appeal among parents with dreams of raising future baseball stars. Playing for the Boston Red Sox from the late 1930s into the 1960s, Ted Williams is regarded as one of Major League Baseball's immortals. He hit 521 home runs, maintained a career batting average of .344, and is the last player to carry a batting average of more than .400 over the course of an entire season. Williams was inducted into his sport's Hall of Fame in 1966. Williams certainly made a prosperous living while playing professional baseball, but he retired from the sport well before salaries exploded in the 1980s and 1990s. Today, a player with the skills of a Ted Williams could command a major league salary that could pay tens of millions of dollars a year.

Experts in genetic science not only found the whole episode unseemly but rather strange as well. After all, it was reported that John Henry Williams had agreed to pay a lab more than $100,000 to keep his father's body frozen—which is a lot more money than one should have to pay to preserve DNA. Indeed, police have been taking tissue and hair samples from suspects in rapes, murders, and assaults for many years in order to perform so-called DNA fingerprinting tests. As part of those tests, labs attempt to match the DNA of the suspect to the DNA found in blood and other evidence unearthed at crime scenes. In such cases, police rarely take more than a tiny slice of tissue or even a few strands of hair from the suspects; DNA is, after all, a molecule, and even the smallest skin sample is likely to contain millions of copies. Once the stories about the fate of the late slugger hit the press, his son dropped out of sight and refused to answer reporters' questions about his motivations for having his father's body frozen.

Ironically, John Henry Williams, who certainly possessed his father's DNA, was never able to take advantage of the genes he inherited from the slugger. John Henry made a brief attempt to forge a baseball career of his own but never made it out of the minor leagues. Moreover, he died of cancer in 2004 and never profited by selling his father's DNA.

Combining the Sciences

For now, reproductive cloning remains fodder for science fiction writers, but many critics worry that science may soon produce methods to create future athletes or geniuses in the test tube. Indeed, concerns about the science of cloning research found their way to the White House in 2009 when President Obama lifted the Bush administration's ban on funding for embryonic stem cell research. As he lifted the ban on stem cell

In March 2009, President Barack Obama signs an executive order lifting the ban on federal funding for embryonic stem cell research. A month later the National Institutes of Health issued guidelines for research on embryos obtained from in vitro fertilization clinics.

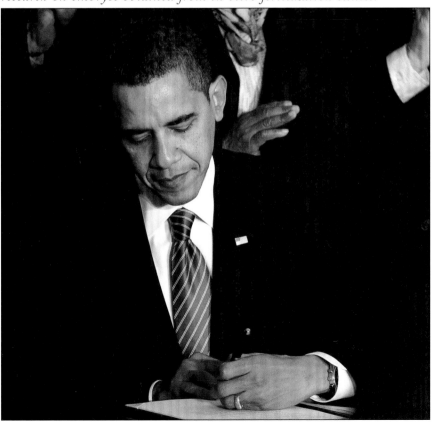

research, the new president declined to rescind the Bush administration's ban on federal funding for therapeutic cloning.

Despite the hesitancy of politicians to support therapeutic cloning as well as some forms of stem cell research, there is no question that both sciences can be combined with gene therapy and that, together, the therapies have the capability of eradicating some truly horrific diseases. There is no clearer example of the potential of combining the sciences than the little girl from Canada who was able to leave the hospital and walk into the sunshine for the first time in her life.

What Is the Future of Gene Therapy?

Since gene therapy is still very much in the experimental phase, the outcomes of many of the therapies under study are not likely to be known for several years. After all, it has been just two decades since Ashanthi DeSilva received new genes to bolster her immune system. It is likely that her health will be monitored closely by gene therapists for many years to come, as they hope to learn much about the reactions of her body over time to the new genes she received as a little girl.

New Gene Therapies

Meanwhile, small steps are constantly being taken at laboratories in America and elsewhere as new gene therapies show the potential of the science. At the University of Washington in Seattle, doctors have taken the first steps toward correcting color blindness through gene therapy. Color blindness affects about 7 percent of American men and about one-half of 1 percent of American women. It is more prevalent among men because the gene that causes the malady is more often found in male chromosomes.

People who are color-blind have difficulty telling the differences between red, yellow, blue, and green. The condition can be more than an annoyance—many color-blind people are unable to drive motor vehicles because they cannot interpret traffic signals. Color blindness is caused by a gene that turns off certain "rods" and "cones"—the cells in the back of the eye that perceive variations of light that transmit colors.

At the University of Washington, scientists injected new genes into the eyes of two color-blind monkeys and soon saw improvement. To test the monkeys, scientists set up an experiment in which the monkeys were prompted to pick colors out of grey dots on a screen. When they touched a colored dot, the monkeys were given sips of juice. After five months of receiving the gene injections, the test animals were consistently picking out the colored dots. Ophthalmology professor Jay Neitz, who headed the study, said that researchers plan to observe the monkeys for an extended period to ensure no ill effects occur and that

CHAPTER FIVE

Turning Off the Aging Gene

Single nucleotide polymorphisms, or SNPs, not only serve as genetic flags for what is wrong with people but can also help doctors understand why some people rarely get sick, recover from illnesses more quickly than others, or even live very long lives. One study conducted in Italy of 52 people who have lived to be 100 or more found a common SNP in 17 percent of the centenarians. When researchers looked for the SNP in 117 people under the age of 99, they found it in only 3 percent of the participants. The researchers concluded that people who possess the SNP in their DNA have four times the chance of living past 100 as those who do not possess the SNP.

Another curious fact was unearthed by the research: Some of the centenarians who possess the SNP were born with it, but others accumulated it through a beneficial genetic mutation that occurred at some point after their births. If scientists can figure out how to duplicate that mutation and make it available to others, they may be able to provide people with opportunities to live past the age of 100. Says Ray Kurzweil, a computer scientist and futurist, "Once we have the ability to change our genes through gene therapy, we will be in a position to turn on genes that promote longevity . . . and turn off those that promote aging."

Ray Kurzweil and Terry Grossman, *Fantastic Voyage*. New York: Plume, 2005, p. 157.

the first human trials may not begin for 10 years or more. Still, Neitz is encouraged by the results. He said, "I have to assume that if we did this exact same thing in a human being today, the human would respond exactly as the monkeys did."[41]

And so it is possible—in the next 10 years or so—that gene replacement therapy will produce a cure for color blindness. Or maybe not. The University of Washington project is typical of gene therapy programs—the research is so new and cutting-edge its outcome remains unknown. Still, given the enthusiasm for the science as well as the billions of dollars in investment that private and public sources are willing to provide, most people involved in genetic science believe that the future will bring new therapies that will undoubtedly ease much suffering and save many lives.

The Search for SNPs

The completion of the human genome map represented the end of a very significant step in the development of gene therapy, but by all measures gene mapping is still very much uncharted territory. The maps that were drawn by the competing public and private projects are general maps of every gene known to exist in the human species. The next step is to map individual patients and base the therapies for their illnesses and disabilities on the specific disease-triggering genes found in their bodies. "This new medical specialty is in its infancy and, as with any new science, there are perils and pitfalls," says Ray Kurzweil, a computer scientist and author of many books that have predicted the future of science. "Today's primitive, incompletely understood tests will lead to ever more sophisticated analyses. Today's magnifying-glass view of the genome will lead to seeing in microscopic detail tomorrow."[42]

As gene mapping becomes more sophisticated, doctors will look for single nucleotide polymorphisms, or SNPs, which are anomalies in the DNA chain. In other words, there are places in the double helix where the adenine, guanine, thymine, or cytosine are out of order. In many cases, SNPs act as biological markers, signaling the location of genes that are associated with diseases. SNPs are not believed to trigger diseases or disabilities, but their presence often suggests that something is wrong in the area of the DNA in which they are found.

The problem, though, is that a DNA chain is estimated to contain as many as 10 million SNPs, which means gene mappers will have to plow through a lot of odd twists and turns in the DNA ladder before they find those that would suggest the presence of disease. Moreover, scientists have already discovered that not all SNPs are bad—some have beneficial qualities. For example, some SNPs have been found in the DNA of people who have survived famines, suggesting that the SNPs in their genetic makeup helped them subsist on a minimal number of calories.

single nucleotide polymorphisms

Points in the DNA chain where the four base chemicals are out of order; also known as SNPs, these anomalies may signal the location of genes associated with diseases.

An important area of research focuses on whether the same SNPs can be found in the same places in the DNA of all patients who have a particular disease or disorder. This area of study is known as "genome-wide associations." In fact, scientists have already managed to identify some SNPs as definitive markers for diabetes, breast cancer, emphysema, high blood pressure (hypertension), and Alzheimer's disease. Tests are available that can identify these SNPs in patients long before they develop those ailments. Some patients can do little with the information but hope they somehow avoid the disease—for example, Alzheimer's disease cannot be cured. But patients who have the SNP that signals high blood pressure can take steps to reduce the likelihood that they will develop hypertension: They can change their diets, lose weight, and exercise. Certainly, a patient with an SNP that indicates the likelihood that he or she will contract the breath-sapping lung disease emphysema would do well to stay away from smoking, smoggy cities, and other environmental triggers of the disease.

The HapMap Project

Helping in the search for SNPs is the International HapMap Project. HapMap stands for haplotype map. When several SNPs cluster together along a DNA strand, they form a haplotype. The HapMap project looks at SNP clusters and examines their roles in inherited diseases among members of specific ethnic groups. Dozens of scientists from Canada, China, Japan, Nigeria, Great Britain, and America have agreed to participate and contribute genetic information they have drawn from members of several races and ethnicities. By 2007 the project had created a haplotype map of some 3 million SNPs.

Working with the HapMap, scientists announced the discovery of an SNP that appears to trigger heart disease in people of European descent. The SNP is so common,

> **haplotype map**
>
> A map of clusters of anomalies in DNA chains that could serve as indicators of diseases.

researchers found, that 50 percent of the European population has inherited it from one parent and 20 percent from both parents. Researchers cautioned, though, that there is no need for half the population of Europe to be alarmed—that to contract heart disease, most would have to observe poor health habits, such as overeating and smoking. And they also pointed out that the SNP may also have a beneficial effect: They reasoned that if the human species, through natural selection, saw no need to rid itself of the SNP over tens of thousands of years of evolution, then the SNP must have a greater purpose than to place people at risk for heart disease. "It is clear that this variant must have some advantage or it couldn't be in 50 percent of the population," said Kari Stefansson, chief executive of DeCode Genetics, a company in Iceland that identified the SNP. "I think it's likely there has been some [reason] for it."[43]

Nanotechnology

The use of DNA to detect the presence of diseases is believed to be so effective that the day may come when X-rays, magnetic resonance imaging scans, mammograms, colonoscopies, and other medical tests are no longer necessary. Some doctors believe it will soon be possible for a patient to simply provide a saliva or blood sample and then, through a DNA analysis performed right in the office, learn whether he or she is likely to contract any number of diseases. To perform the DNA analyses, doctors may make use of nanotechnology, which employs tiny particles or devices—100 nanometers or smaller. A nanometer is a billionth of a meter.

> **nanotechnology**
>
> The use of tiny particles or devices, no larger than a few billionths of a meter, to study molecules or alter their functions.

At Harvard University, researchers have already developed a device that makes use of nanotechnology in the form of nanowires, which are tiny silicon wires. The wires can detect genes in the blood that are known to trigger prostate cancer—when the wires come into contact with one of the genetic triggers they spark an electrical signal. The nanowires used in the prostate cancer experiment are 10 nanometers, or 10 billionths of a meter, in width.

"This is one of the first applications of nanotechnology to healthcare and offers a clinical technique that is significantly better than what exists today," says the developer of the device, Harvard chemistry professor Charles M. Lieber. "A nanowire array can test a mere pinprick of blood in just minutes, providing a nearly instantaneous scan for many different cancer markers. It's a device that could open up substantial new possibilities in the diagnosis of cancer and other complex diseases."[44] Currently, the common tests for prostate cancer include a rectal examination by a physician, who probes for an enlargement of the prostate gland, followed by a blood test that screens for a protein common in prostate cancer cases. It often takes a week or more before the results of the blood test are known.

Synthetic Biology and *Jurassic Park*

The novel *Jurassic Park* and its film version suggest that it is possible to clone dinosaurs by implanting their DNA into frog embryos. By using synthetic biology, scientists at Pennsylvania State University believe cloning prehistoric beasts can be more than just science fiction.

In this case, the scientists say they can replicate a wooly mammoth, an elephant-like creature that has been extinct for 10,000 years. The scientists have been able to extract DNA from a tuft of mammoth hair and map most of the beast's genome. They propose using synthetic biology to fill in some 400,000 gaps in the mammoth's genome by using pieces of DNA from modern-day elephants. Theoretically, they could build their own wooly mammoth DNA molecule, inject it into an elephant embryo, implant the embryo into a female elephant and then await the birth of a wooly mammoth, the first in about 10,000 years. At this point, the only obstacle standing in the way of cloning a new wooly mammoth is money—the Penn State researchers lack the $10 million they predict it would cost to carry out the experiment. Says biochemistry professor Stephan C. Schuster, "This is something that could work, though it will be tedious and expensive."

Quoted in Nicholas Wade, "Regenerating a Mammoth for $10 Million," *New York Times*, November 20, 2008, p. A-1.

Biobots

Nanotechnology has been combined with gene therapy in other ways. At Emory University in Georgia, scientists have developed nanoparticles known as quantum dots that are about the size of a molecule. These nanoparticles glow when they come into contact with certain genes or proteins, meaning they can be used to identify the proteins common in cancerous cells. And if quantum dots can be used to identify genetic triggers of diseases, many gene therapists believe they can also be used to deliver drugs to shut down genes that trigger diseases. These devices are known as biobots. Essentially, a biobot would be a tiny robot programmed to deliver the drug to a gene and shut down the gene or otherwise fix what is wrong with its DNA. At this point, biobots are still theoretical, but many scientists see the likelihood of their development in the next few years. Says Robert A. Freitas Jr., a senior research fellow at the Institute for Molecular Manufacturing in Palo Alto, California, "Artificial biobots could be in our bodies in the next five to ten years. Advances in genetic engineering are likely to allow us to construct an artificial microbe . . . to perform certain functions. These biobots could be designed to produce vitamins, hormones [or] enzymes . . . in which the host body was deficient, or they could be programmed to selectively absorb and break down poisons and toxins."[45]

BioBricks and Synthetic Biology

One of the most cutting-edge uses of genetic science under development is known as synthetic biology. Essentially, the science involves taking pieces of DNA from a number of sources and putting them together to form a new organism. Each piece of DNA is regarded as a building block; in fact, the pieces are known as BioBricks. Scientists compare them to the plastic bricks found in a child's LEGO set.

While it would seem that by using synthetic biology scientists could eventually engineer a living and breathing creature of their own design, such notions are reserved for science fiction writers. At this point, scientists see synthetic biology as a method of reengineering bacteria and other very simple organisms that, nevertheless, could make a deep impact on medical science.

Indeed, synthetic biology has enormous potential for eradicating horrific diseases. Already, BioBricks have been used to manufacture a drug that will be used to combat malaria. The drug is under development and expected to be administered to patients by 2012.

Malaria kills up to a million people a year, mostly children living in the tropics. It is spread by mosquitoes that bite their victims, injecting microscopic disease-carrying parasites into their blood. The standard treatment for malaria is a drug in which the active ingredient is the chemical chloroquine. Starting in the 1990s, though, doctors noticed that some malaria patients had stopped responding to their chloroquine treatments. Evidently, the parasite had built up a resistance to chloroquine, which is a typical development in the evolution of some diseases.

Scientists have found a substitute for chloroquine: the chemical artemisinin, which can be extracted from a wildflower known as sweet

quantum dots

About the size of a molecule, a particle that glows when it comes into contact with certain genes or proteins; useful in identifying the proteins common in cancerous cells.

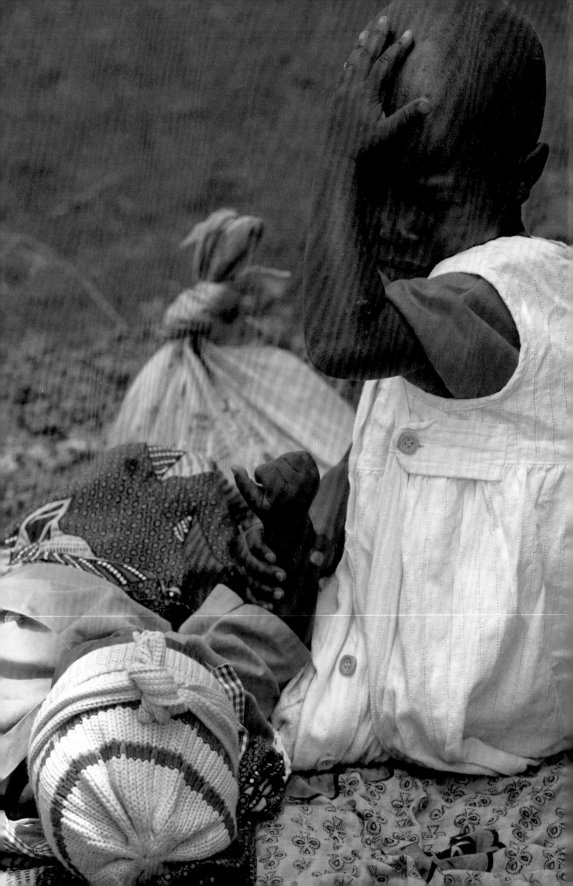

A young boy holds his sister's hand as she awaits treatment for malaria at a hospital in Kenya. Some patients do not respond to traditional malaria drugs. Research in synthetic biology, a new branch of genetic science, may lead to more-effective malaria drugs.

wormwood. (The scientific name of the plant is *Artemisia annua*). The problem, though, is that sweet wormwood is not a cultivated plant—it grows in the wild. To mass-produce a drug composed of artemisinin, farms would have to devote thousands of acres to growing sweet wormwood while factories gear up to extract the drug from the plant. It could take many years before a sweet wormwood crop is big enough to provide enough artemisinin to fulfill the needs of a widespread malaria treatment program. In the meantime, the lives of millions of people are at risk.

Moving Research into the Real World

By employing synthetic biology, scientists at the University of California at Berkeley have stepped in to provide hope. They have been able to produce artemisinin in the test tube by cobbling together pieces of DNA from other sources to reproduce the genome of the sweet wormwood plant. Next, they inserted their handmade genes into an *E. coli* bacterium, which then went through the natural process of cell reproduction. In other words, the Berkeley scientists had started their own artemisinin factory but without the need for thousands of acres to grow a crop of sweet wormwood. "Making a few micrograms of artemisinin would have been a neat scientific trick," says Jay Keasling, the Berkeley biochemical engineer who heads

> **biobots**
>
> Tiny devices that might one day be used to deliver drugs to a faulty gene, shutting down the gene or otherwise fixing what is wrong with its DNA.

the project, "but it doesn't do anybody in Africa any good if all we can do is a cool experiment in a Berkeley lab. We need to make it on an industrial scale."[46]

The technology developed by the Berkeley scientists has been made available to drug companies, which are now gearing up to provide artemisinin-based antimalaria drugs to patients in Africa and other tropical locations. Meanwhile, given their success in producing artemisinin in a test tube, the scientists are convinced that the techniques can be employed to manufacture other drugs. Says Keasling, "We ought to be able to make any compound produced by a plant inside a microbe. We ought to have all these metabolic pathways. You need this drug: OK, we pull this piece, this part, and this one off the shelf. You put them into a microbe, and two weeks later out comes your product."[47]

Exciting Possibilities

The production of artemisinin in a test tube is possible because the scientists at Berkeley were able to map the genome of sweet wormwood. Mapping the human genome is, of course, much more complicated. When, as Kurzweil predicts, every person will have his or her genome individually mapped, the next step will be to store those maps on microchips or even CD-ROMs. When people feel ill, they will take their CD-ROM to the doctor who will put it into a computer and provide a diagnosis based partially on the information contained on the disk. If, for example, the doctor hears an abnormal heartbeat, he or she will know which genes may be the culprits and then check the CD-ROM to see if that patient carries those genes. Likewise, the therapy prescribed by the doctor will not be as it often is now—to treat the symptoms—but rather to completely eradicate the problem by fixing the faulty gene.

More important, though, Kurzweil says that people will know at very early ages whether they carry genes that could trigger certain diseases, particularly cancers. Armed with such information, he says, people can then take steps to avoid foods or environments that would increase their chances of developing the type of cancerous tumors that may be prompted by the foods they eat or the type of air they breathe. He says, "You [will] have the ability to both know and modify the expression of the genes you were born with through diet, nutrition, and lifestyle choices."[48]

synthetic biology

The use of DNA from other sources to engineer new organisms that can be useful in manufacturing drugs unavailable through conventional methods.

Gene therapy and its associated sciences have emerged as exciting and challenging branches of medicine. As the cases of Ashanthi DeSilva and Katlyn Demerchant illustrate, gene therapy can save the lives of

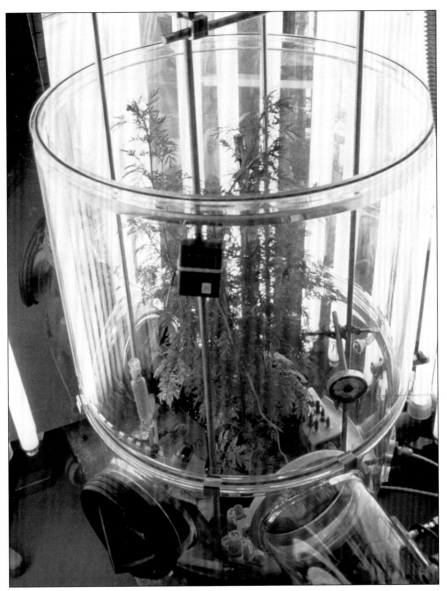

Sweet wormwood, sealed in a glass growth chamber, is being studied as the source of a chemical that is useful in treating malaria. Gene researchers are working on ways to produce that chemical in large quantities.

young children. For Steven Howarth, gene therapy has ensured that he will continue to have the use of his eyes. Meanwhile, Chrissy Falletti waits for a cure for cystic fibrosis while Louise Cooper climbs mountains and lives a full life thanks to a genetically engineered drug that eradicated a cancer-causing protein in her body.

An End to Suffering

But genetic research is likely to proceed slowly because of its unknown consequences. Certainly, no one involved in the science wants to see the mistakes repeated that cost the life of Jesse Gelsinger. And while tremendous benefits may be realized through animal pharming and therapeutic cloning, the ethical and social implications of those sciences may raise doubts among many people who, ultimately, may choose other therapies that do not include an acceptance of drugs produced by animals or cures developed by tinkering with the DNA of an embryo. It would seem, though, that there will be plenty of time to resolve many of those issues. In the meantime, genetic research continues to provide amazing results, giving hope to people who suffer from truly horrific diseases.

Source Notes

Introduction: Replacing Faulty Genes

1. Quoted in Laura Blue, "A Gene to Cure Blindness," *Time*, May 18, 2007. www.time.com.

2. Jeff Lyon and Peter Gorner, *Altered Fates: Gene Therapy and the Retooling of Human Life*. New York: W.W. Norton, 1995, p. 29.

3. Horace Freeland Judson, "The Glimmering Promise of Gene Therapy," *Technology Review*, November/December 2006, p. 42.

4. Quoted in Blue, "A Gene to Cure Blindness."

Chapter One: What Is Gene Therapy?

5. Quoted in Lyon and Gorner, *Altered Fates*, p. 31.

6. Lyon and Gorner, *Altered Fates*, p. 13.

7. Quoted in Nathan Sheppard, ed., *Darwinism Stated by Darwin Himself*. New York: Appleton, 1884, p. 68.

8. Quoted in Sheppard, *Darwinism Stated by Darwin Himself*, p. 69.

9. Quoted in Walter Bodmer and Robin McKie, *The Book of Man: The Human Genome Project and the Quest to Discover Our Genetic Heritage*. New York: Scribner, 1994, p. 31.

10. Quoted in Ivan Noble, "'Secret of Life' Discovery Turns 50," BBC News, February 27, 2003. http://news.bbc.co.uk.

11. Quoted in Ramez Naam, "More than Human," *New York Times*, July 3, 2005. www.nytimes.com.

12. Quoted in Lyon and Gorner, *Altered Fates*, p. 239.

13. Quoted in PBS *NewsHour*, "Gene Therapy," December 8, 1999. www.pbs.org.

14. Quoted in Karen Springen, "Using Genes as Medicine," *Newsweek*, December 6, 2004, p. 55.

15. Quoted in PBS *NewsHour*, "Sequencing Life," February 12, 2001. www.pbs.org.

16. Quoted in PBS *NewsHour*, "Sequencing Life."

Chapter Two: The Ideal Gene-Delivery Vehicle: Viruses

17. Quoted in PBS *NewsHour*, "Gene Therapy," December 8, 1999. www.pbs.org.

18. Quoted in Leon Jaroff and Alice Park, "Fixing the Genes," *Time*, January 11, 1999, p. 68.

19. Quoted in Jaroff and Park, "Fixing the Genes," p. 68.

20. Quoted in Marie McCullough, "Apology for Study That Left Teen Dead," *Philadelphia Inquirer*, May 8, 2009, p. A-1.

21. Paul Gelsinger, "Seeking Justice for My Son," *Philadelphia Inquirer*, September 17, 2009, p. A-11.

22. Quoted in McCullough, "Apology for Study That Left Teen Dead," p. A-1.

23. Quoted in Andrew Pollack, "Cancer Risk Exceeds Outlook in Gene Therapy, Studies Find," *New York Times*, June 13, 2003, p. A-29.

24. Quoted in Larry Thompson, "Human Gene Therapy," *FDA Consumer*, September/October 2000, p. 19.

25. Quoted in Sarah Webb, "Cellular Smugglers," *Science News*, June 30, 2007, p. 404.

Chapter Three: Attacking Bad Genes with Drugs

26. Bodmer and McKie, *The Book of Man: The Human Genome Project and the Quest to Discover Our Genetic Heritage*, p. 240.

27. Quoted in BBC News, "Trial Drugs 'Reverse' Alzheimer's," May 6, 2009. http://news.bbc.co.uk.

28. Quoted in Jerome Goopman, "Open Channels: Do New Cystic Fibrosis Therapies Hold the Key to Treating Other Genetic Disorders?" *New Yorker*, May 4, 2009, p. 30.

29. Quoted in Goopman, "Open Channels," p. 31.

30. Quoted in Liz Szabo, "A New Age in Cancer Care: In 10 Years, Breakout Drug Herceptin Has Led Way in Targeting Breast Tumors," *USA Today*, October 13, 2008, p. D-5.

31. Quoted in David G. Nathan, "Ken's Story: One Patient's Role in the Cancer Treatment Revolution," *Harvard Magazine*, January/February 2007, p. 46.

32. Quoted in Andrew Pollack, "Patient's DNA May Be Signal to Tailor Drugs," *New York Times*, December 30, 2008, p. A-1.

33. Quoted in Alla Katsnelson, "A Drug to Call One's Own: Will Medicine Finally Get Personal?" *Scientific American*, August 1, 2005. www.scientificamerican.com.

34. David G. Nathan, "The Amazing Power of an Experimental Cancer Drug Gave One Patient Three Years of Life and a New Mission," *Boston Globe*, March 12, 2007, p. C-1.

Chapter Four: Stem Cells, Cloning, and Gene Therapy

35. Quoted in Jill Neimark, "The DNA Cure," *Discover*, September 2009, p. 36.

36. Quoted in New York Presbyterian Hospital–Weill Cornel Medical Center news release, "Gene Therapy Could Expand Stem Cells' Promise," May 21, 2009. http://news.med.cornell.edu.

37. Quoted in *Scientist*, "Patched-Up Human Stem Cells," May 31, 2009. www.the-scientist.com.

38. Leon R. Kass and James Q. Wilson, *The Ethics of Human Cloning*. Washington: AEI Press, 1998, p. 17.

39. Quoted in Alice Park, "The Perils of Cloning," *Time*, July 5, 2006. www.time.com.

40. Quoted in Tom Verducci and Lester Munson, "What Really Happened to Ted Williams?" *Sports Illustrated*, August 18, 2003, p. 66.

Chapter Five: What Is the Future of Gene Therapy?

41. Quoted in Jeanna Bryner, "Gene Therapy Lets Monkeys See in Color," September 16, 2009. LiveScience. http://news.aol.com.

42. Ray Kurzweil and Terry Grossman, *Fantastic Voyage*. New York: Plume, 2005, p. 159.

43. Quoted in Nicholas Wade, "Gene Called Predictor of Heart Disease Risk; Scientists Say Telltale Variation Common Among Those of European Blood," *Albany (NY) Times Union*, May 4, 2007, p. A-1.

44. Quoted in Medical News Today, "Nanowires for Detecting Molecular Signs of Cancer," September 24, 2005. www.medicalnewstoday.com.

45. Quoted in Kurzweil and Grossman, *Fantastic Voyage*, p. 155.

46. Quoted in Michael Specter, "A Life of Its Own: Where Will Synthetic Biology Lead Us?" *New Yorker*, September 28, 2009, p. 58.

47. Quoted in Specter, "A Life of Its Own," p. 59.

48. Kurzweil and Grossman, *Fantastic Voyage*, p. 159.

Facts About Gene Therapy

DNA

- One chromosome can contain as little as 50 million and as many as 250 million pairs of the four DNA base chemicals adenine, thymine, cytosine, and guanine.

- The human body contains about 3 billion DNA molecules.

- If one were to unwind all the DNA found in all the cells of one person and link the strands end to end, the chain would be long enough to reach the moon 6,000 times.

- The private company Celera Genomics, which mapped the human genome, based its research on DNA collected from five volunteers.

- The DNA double helix molecule resembles a twisting ladder; in almost everyone, the ladder twists to the right.

- Everyone's DNA is 99.8 percent similar, meaning that regardless of height, weight, gender, race, and ethnicity, the chemical makeup of all people on Earth differs by only two tenths of 1 percent.

- About 97 percent of the DNA found in humans has no known function.

The Human Genome

- When scientists started mapping the human genome in 1990 they expected to find more than 100,000 genes; instead, the final total is about 23,000.

- The publicly funded project to map the human genome cost about $3 billion over the course of 13 years.

- Drug companies pay about $8 million a year for access to the gene map composed by Celera Genomics.

- There are about 19,000 genes in roundworms, 13,000 in fruit flies, about 6,000 in yeast, and about 4,000 found in the germ that causes tuberculosis.

- The DNA found in the human and chimpanzee genomes differs by only 2 percent.

- Since 2007, various projects have been established to map the genomes of individuals—about 1,000 people in total are having their DNA mapped in these projects.

- The goal of the Personal Genome Project at Harvard University is to map the genomes of 100,000 people.

- Seven percent of the human genome has changed within the past 5,000 to 10,000 years.

Diseases Caused by Faulty Genes

- Most people are born with 46 chromosomes—23 inherited from each parent. Down syndrome patients are born with an extra, or forty-seventh, chromosome.

- Turner syndrome, which afflicts only girls, manifests itself in dwarfism, failure to reach puberty, learning disabilities, and heart defects and is caused by the patient having inherited 23 chromosomes from one parent and 22 from the other.

- Nine of the 10 leading causes of death in America, among them heart disease, cancer, and diabetes, are caused by diseases sparked by faulty or mutated genes.

- About 100 diseases that cause blindness are sparked by the failure of a single gene.

- Genes can mutate during a person's lifetime due to a variety of causes, such as exposure to drugs, chemicals, or ultraviolet radiation from sunlight.

Genetics Research

- Since Ashanthi DeSilva received new genes in 1990, about 4,000 patients have participated in gene therapy trials.

- The National Institutes of Health provides more than $400 million a year to projects studying gene therapy.

- Laboratories are able to test for about 1,000 faulty genes that are known to cause various diseases and debilitations.

- By genetically altering the *E. coli* bacteria, students at the Massachusetts Institute of Technology have found a way to give the foul-smelling germ the aroma of wintergreen mint.

Cloning

- Dolly, the first sheep conceived through reproductive cloning, died of lung cancer at the age of six. She also had arthritis.

- More than 90 percent of attempts to reproduce animals or other organisms through reproductive cloning fail.

- Typically, it takes some 100 attempts to transfer the nucleus of a cell into an egg to carry out the cloning process.

- A study of 10,000 liver and placenta cells of cloned mice found that 4 percent of their genes were abnormal.

Related Organizations

American Enterprise Institute (AEI)
1150 17th St. NW
Washington, DC 20036
phone: (202) 862-5800
fax: (202) 862-7177
Web site: www.aei.org

The organization opposes the science of reproductive cloning, suggesting that it could lead to the unnatural development of children with superior intellects or athletic abilities. Students can download copies of the book *The Ethics of Human Cloning* by AEI scholars Leon R. Kass and James Q. Wilson.

Center for Bioethics and Culture
130 Market Pl., No. 146
San Ramon, CA 94583
Web Site: www.cbc-network.org

The Center for Bioethics and Culture supports gene therapy and stem cell research. Visitors to the organization's Web site can find essays about genetic research and download news articles and other materials about gene therapy, stem cell research, cloning, eugenics, and similar issues.

Center for Genetics and Society
1936 University Ave., Suite 350
Berkeley, CA 94704
phone: (510) 625-0819
fax: (510) 625-0874
e-mail: info@geneticsandsociety.org
Web site: www.geneticsandsociety.org

The center supports the study of therapeutic cloning as well as stem cell research. Young people can find many resources about therapeutic cloning and similar issues by accessing the "For Students" link on the organization's Web site, including a background on genetic diagnoses as well as many lists of frequently asked questions about cloning.

Cystic Fibrosis Foundation
6931 Arlington Rd.
Bethesda, MD 20814
phone: (800) 344-4823
fax: (301) 951-6378
e-mail: info@cff.org
Web site: www.cff.org

The Cystic Fibrosis Foundation raises money to fund research into cystic fibrosis, which is caused by a faulty gene. By accessing the link on the organization's Web site for "Research Overview," students can read about how gene therapy is employed to develop new medications and other therapies to treat cystic fibrosis.

National Human Genome Research Institute
National Institutes of Health
Bldg. 31, Room 4B09
31 Center Dr., MSC 2152
9000 Rockville Pike
Bethesda, MD 20892-2152
phone: (301) 402-0911
fax: (301) 402-2218
Web site: www.genome.gov

The National Genome Research Institute headed the federal government's project to map the human genome. Visitors to the agency's Web site can read an overview of the project and how the genome map is assisting gene therapy researchers. The Web site also includes an archive of information on the discovery and characteristics of DNA.

Parkinson's Disease Foundation
1359 Broadway, Suite 1509
New York, NY 10018
phone: (212) 923-4700
fax: (212) 923-4778
Web site: www.pdf.org

The Parkinson's Disease Foundation raises money to fund research projects aimed at wiping out the neurological disease. By entering "gene therapy" into the search engine on the foundation's Web site, students can find many news articles and research reports on the gene therapy projects funded by the foundation.

Synthetic Biology Project

Woodrow Wilson International Center for Scholars
One Woodrow Wilson Plaza
1300 Pennsylvania Ave. NW
Washington, DC 20004-3027
phone: (202) 691-4320
fax: (202) 691-4001
e-mail: synbio@wilsoncenter.org
Web site: www.synbioproject.org

The Synthetic Biology Project provides a number of resources about the science of synthetic biology, which employs DNA to construct new organisms. The project has made a number of resources available on its Web site focusing on the science behind synthetic biology as well as the ethical issues that surround the science.

U.S. Food and Drug Administration (FDA)

5600 Fishers Ln.
Rockville, MD 20857-0001
phone: (888) 463-6332
Web site: www.fda.gov

The FDA monitors all gene therapy trials in America. Students can find many resources about gene therapy and the nature of many trials that are under way at the FDA's Cellular and Gene Therapy Products Web site.

For Further Research

Books

Andrea L. Bonnicksen, *Chimeras, Hybrids, and Interspecies Research: Politics and Policymaking*. Washington, DC: Georgetown University Press, 2009.

Molly Fitzgerald-Hayes and Frieda Reichsman, *DNA and Biotechnology*. Burlington, MA: Academic Press, 2009.

Jonathan Kimmelman, *Gene Transfer and the Ethics of First-in-Human Research: Lost in Translation*. New York: Cambridge University Press, 2009.

Paul J.H. Schoemaker and Joyce A. Schoemaker, *Chips, Clones, and Living Beyond 100: How Far Will the Biosciences Take Us?* Upper Saddle River, NJ: FT Press, 2009.

Spencer S. Stober and Donna Yarri, *God, Science, and Designer Genes: An Exploration of Emerging Genetic Technologies*. Santa Barbara, CA: Praeger, 2009.

Periodicals

Jerome Goopman, "Open Channels: Do New Cystic Fibrosis Therapies Hold the Key to Treating Other Genetic Disorders?" *New Yorker*, May 4, 2009, p. 30.

David G. Nathan, "The Amazing Power of an Experimental Cancer Drug Gave One Patient Three Years of Life and a New Mission," *Boston Globe*, March 12, 2007, p. C-1.

Jill Neimark, "The DNA Cure," *Discover*, September 2009, p. 36.

Delthia Ricks, "Gene Therapy May Help Patients Get Their Lives Back," *Newsday*, June 22, 2007, p. A-17.

Michael Specter, "A Life of Its Own: Where Will Synthetic Biology Lead Us?" *New Yorker*, September 28, 2009, p. 58.

Web Sites

Genetics Home Reference, "What Is Gene Therapy?" (http://ghr.nlm. nih.gov/handbook/therapy/genetherapy). This site, maintained by the National Library of Medicine, allows students to download a 146-page handbook titled *Help Me Understand Genetics*. The book includes chapters on cells and DNA, how genes function, mutations, how genes are inherited, genetic testing, gene therapy, and other issues.

Medline Plus, "Genes and Gene Therapy" (www.nlm.nih.gov/med lineplus/genesandgenetherapy.html). Maintained by the National Institutes of Health, the Web site explains the background of gene therapy and its application for treating many genetically caused diseases and debilitations.

On Being a Scientist: A Guide to Responsible Conduct in Research (www.nap.edu/openbook.php?record_id=12192&page=R1). This is a free, downloadable book from the National Academy of Sciences Committee on Science, Engineering, and Public Policy. The 2009 edition provides a clear explanation of the responsible conduct of scientific research. Chapters on treatment of data, mistakes and negligence, the scientist's role in society, and other topics offer invaluable insight for student researchers.

PBS, "Genetic Research: A Health Spotlight Focus" (www.pbs.org/news hour/bb/health/july-dec99/gene_therapy_splash.htm). The companion Web site to the PBS *NewsHour* series on gene therapy covers such issues as mapping the human genome, the therapy that saved the life of Ashanthi DeSilva, and the experiment that led to the death of Jesse Gelsinger.

***Time* Collection, "Cloning"** (www.time.com/time/archive/collections/ 0,21428,c_cloning,00.shtml). *Time* magazine has established an extensive archive of its articles on reproductive and therapeutic cloning. Students can find *Time* cover stories on human cloning research, stem cell research, Dolly the cloned sheep, and the DNA mapping projects.

University of Utah, Genetic Science Learning Center, "Gene Therapy: Molecular Bandage?" (http://learn.genetics.utah.edu/content/tech/ genetherapy). This Web site explains gene therapy and how researchers select the genetically caused diseases to attack. The site includes an extensive explanation of what causes cystic fibrosis and how gene therapy is seeking a cure to the disease.

Index.

proteomics, 17

quantum dots, 72, 73

radiation therapy, 50
red blood cells, normal *vs.* sickle-
  cell, 23 (illustration)
Repoxugen, 49
reproductive cloning, 56, 60–62,
  64
research
  on embryonic stem cells,
    support for, 57
  on gene replacement therapy for
    color blindness, 67–68
  in gene therapy, complexity of,
    13–14
Rhucin, 52
ribonucleic acid (RNA), 20–21,
  24
Robinson, Harriet L., 34

Sanger, Frederick, 21
Schuster, Stephan C., 72
severe combined
  immunodeficiency (SCID), 22
  stem cell therapy in, 54–55
Shaw, George Bernard, 56
sickle-cell anemia, 20
  early research on, 19–20
single nucleotide polymorphisms
  (SNPs), 68, 69–70
  haplotype maps of, 70–71
smart drugs, 42
  development of, 45–47
somatic cell nuclear transfer
  (SCNT), 58–59
Springstein, Thomas, 49
Stefansson, Kari, 71
stem cells
  adult, 58

differentiation of, 60
  embryonic, 56–57
  in treatment of severe combined
    immunodeficiency, 54–55
  undifferentiated nature of, 55
stem cell therapy, combination
  with gene therapy, 57–58
stomach cancer, 49–50
surveys, on support for embryonic
  stem cell research, 57
synthetic biology, 73, 75, 76

tamoxifen, 48
Tay-Sachs disease, 20
therapeutic cloning, 60, 62
  See also somatic cell nuclear
    transfer
Time (magazine), 57
transgenic animals, 50

undifferentiated stem cells, 55
Uslan, Jody, 47–48

vectors, 30
  bacteria as, 39
  liposomes as, 38–39
  viruses as, 29–32
Vetter, David, 22
viruses
  as vectors of genes, 29–32
    risks of, 32, 34–38
  workings of, 33 (illustration)

Watson, James D., 21, 27, 41
Williams, John Henry, 64–65
Williams, Ted, 62, 64
Wilmut, Ian, 62
Wilson, James M., 32, 35, 36
Wood, Rebecca, 42

xenotransplantation, 44

94

Picture Credits

Cover: iStockphoto.com
Maury Aaseng: 33, 59
AP Images: 11, 65, 74
iStockphoto.com: 8, 9, 37, 43
Photoshot: 51, 65
Science Photo Library: 16, 18, 23, 27, 46, 63, 77

About the Author

Hal Marcovitz has written more than 150 books for young readers. A former daily newspaper reporter and columnist, he makes his home in Chalfont, Pennsylvania, with his wife Gail and daughter Ashley. As a journalist, Marcovitz is a three-time winner of the Keystone Press Award, the Pennsylvania Newspaper Association's highest award for journalism. His 2005 biography of U.S. House Speaker Nancy Pelosi was named to *Booklist* magazine's list of recommended feminist books for young readers. He also served as chief writer and associate editor for *Taught to Lead,* an anthology of essays chronicling the educations of the presidents of the United States, and is co-author of *Bloom's Literary Places: Rome,* a traveler's guide to places in Rome where famous writers such as F. Scott Fitzgerald, Tennessee Williams and Gore Vidal lived and worked. Marcovitz is also the author of the comic novel *Painting the White House.*

ABOUT THE AUTHOR